# Lecture Notes in Computer Science    15408

Founding Editors

Gerhard Goos
Juris Hartmanis

The series Lecture Notes in Computer Science (LNCS), including its subseries Lecture Notes in Artificial Intelligence (LNAI) and Lecture Notes in Bioinformatics (LNBI), has established itself as a medium for the publication of new developments in computer science and information technology research, teaching, and education.

LNCS enjoys close cooperation with the computer science R & D community, the series counts many renowned academics among its volume editors and paper authors, and collaborates with prestigious societies. Its mission is to serve this international community by providing an invaluable service, mainly focused on the publication of conference and workshop proceedings and postproceedings. LNCS commenced publication in 1973.

Ruisheng Su · Ezequiel de la Rosa ·
Leonhard Rist · Ewout Heylen ·
Frank te Nijenhuis · Danny Ruijters ·
Markus D. Schirmer · Richard McKinley ·
Susanne Wegener · Roland Wiest ·
Theo van Walsum
Editors

# Image Analysis in Stroke Diagnosis and Interventions

4th International Workshop, SWITCH 2024
and 6th International Challenge, ISLES 2024
Held in Conjunction with MICCAI 2024
Marrakesh, Morocco, October 10, 2024
Proceedings

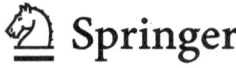

*Editors*
Ruisheng Su [ID]
Eindhoven University of Technology
Eindhoven, The Netherlands

Ezequiel de la Rosa
University of Zurich
Zurich, Switzerland

Leonhard Rist
Friedrich-Alexander-Universität
Erlangen, Germany

Ewout Heylen [ID]
KU Leuven
Leuven, Belgium

Frank te Nijenhuis
Erasmus MC
Rotterdam, The Netherlands

Danny Ruijters
Eindhoven University of Technology
Eindhoven, The Netherlands

Markus D. Schirmer [ID]
Massachusetts General Hospital
Boston, MA, USA

Richard McKinley
University Hospital Inselspital
Bern, Switzerland

Susanne Wegener
University Hospital Zurich
Zurich, Switzerland

Roland Wiest
University Hospital Inselspital
Bern, Switzerland

Theo van Walsum [ID]
Erasmus MC
Rotterdam, The Netherlands

ISSN 0302-9743      ISSN 1611-3349  (electronic)
Lecture Notes in Computer Science
ISBN 978-3-031-81100-5      ISBN 978-3-031-81101-2  (eBook)
https://doi.org/10.1007/978-3-031-81101-2

This Springer imprint is published by the registered company Springer Nature Switzerland AG
The registered company address is: Gewerbestrasse 11, 6330 Cham, Switzerland

If disposing of this product, please recycle the paper.

# Contents

## ISLES

# SWITCH

# Preface

This volume comprises articles from the Stroke Workshop on Imaging and Treatment Challenges (SWITCH 2024) and the Ischemic Stroke Lesion Segmentation Challenge (ISLES 2024). These events were held as an integrated program in conjunction with the Medical Image Computing and Computer Assisted Intervention (MICCAI) conference from October 6th to 10th, 2024, in Marrakesh, Morocco.

The manuscripts presented herein describe research advancements in image analysis for the diagnosis and intervention of ischemic and haemorrhagic stroke. While this compilation does not claim to provide a comprehensive understanding from all perspectives, it presents some of the latest developments in segmentation, disease prognosis, stroke diagnosis and treatment, and other clinically relevant applications.

The volume is divided into two chapters. The first chapter contains the eight accepted papers out of twelve valid submissions to the SWITCH workshop track of the integrated event. The review process was double-blinded, with at least two reviewers followed by one meta-review. The second chapter includes four papers submitted and accepted to the ISLES track, which describe the solutions submitted to the ISLES challenge. These four papers were reviewed in a single-blinded manner by one reviewer followed by one meta-reviewer.

The **first chapter** focuses on imaging related to stroke diagnosis and treatment. The main objectives of the workshop were: 1) to introduce the clinical background of challenges and opportunities related to stroke imaging that are relevant to researchers in the MICCAI community, and 2) to stimulate discussion and the exchange of ideas. The workshop featured keynote presentations by clinical experts in stroke imaging and treatment, along with presentations of accepted works by participating authors. In this edition, Robin Lemmens from KU Leuven delivered a keynote addressing the role of medical imaging in current and future stroke care practices. The topics addressed in the accepted papers were presented in two subsections: 1) AI applications in stroke, and 2) stroke lesion segmentation methods.

The **second chapter** presents a selection of papers from participants in the ISLES 2024 challenge. The ISLES challenge focused on image-based clinical decision support for the treatment of ischemic stroke patients, emphasizing the accurate estimation of core (irreversibly damaged tissue) and penumbra (salvageable tissue) volumes. In this edition, the challenge centered on predicting the temporal evolution of the core from acute imaging data, which is crucial for clinical decision-making. Understanding the growth rate of the core is vital for assessing the feasibility of transferring a patient to a comprehensive stroke center, especially considering transport times. Moreover, since not all reperfusion treatments with mechanical thrombectomy result in complete reperfusion, predicting infarct growth may provide interventional radiologists with insights into the potential benefits of additional reperfusion attempts.

The organizers of SWITCH and ISLES extend their sincere gratitude to the keynote speaker, the contributing authors, and the workshop attendees. The organizers sincerely hope that this volume will inspire further exciting research advances in stroke image analysis in and beyond MICCAI.

November 2024

Ewout Heylen
Richard McKinley
Frank te Nijenhuis
Leonhard Rist
Ezequiel de la Rosa
Danny Ruijters
Markus D. Schirmer
Ruisheng Su
Theo van Walsum
Susanne Wegener
Roland Wiest

# From Diagnostic CT to DTI Tractography Labels: Using Deep Learning for Corticospinal Tract Injury Assessment and Outcome Prediction in Intracerebral Haemorrhage

Olivia N Murray[1]([✉]), Hamied Haroon[1], Paul Ryu[2], Hiren Patel[3], Geroge Harston[4], Marieke Wermer[5], Wilmar Jolink[6], Daniel Hanley[2], Catharina Klijn[7], Ulrike Hammerbeck[8], Adrian Parry-Jones[1], and Timothy Cootes[1]

[1] University of Manchester, Manchester, UK
olivia.murray@manchester.ac.uk
[2] Johns Hopkins, Baltimore, USA
[3] Salford Royal NHS Foundation Trust, Salford, UK
[4] Brainomix, Oxford, UK
[5] Leiden University, Leiden, The Netherlands
[6] Isala Zwolle, Zwolle, The Netherlands
[7] Radboud University Medical Centre, Nijmegen, The Netherlands
[8] King's College London, London, UK

**Abstract.** The preservation of the corticospinal tract (CST) is key to good motor recovery after stroke. The gold standard method of assessing the CST with imaging is diffusion tensor tractography. However, this is not available for most intracerebral haemorrhage (ICH) patients. Non-contrast CT scans are routinely available in most ICH diagnostic pipelines, but delineating white matter from a CT scan is challenging. We utilise nnU-Net, trained on paired diagnostic CT scans and high-directional diffusion tractography maps, to segment the CST from diagnostic CT scans alone, and we show our model reproduces diffusion based tractography maps of the CST with a Dice similarity coefficient of 57%.

Surgical haematoma evacuation is sometimes performed after ICH, but published clinical trials to date show that whilst surgery reduces mortality, there is no evidence of improved functional recovery. Restricting surgery to patients with an intact CST may reveal a subset of patients for whom haematoma evacuation improves functional outcome. We investigated the clinical utility of our model in the MISTIE III clinical trial dataset. We found that our model's CST integrity measure significantly predicted outcome after ICH in the acute and chronic time frames, therefore providing a prognostic marker for patients to whom advanced diffusion tensor imaging is unavailable. This will allow for future probing of subgroups who may benefit from surgery.

**Keywords:** DWI and Tractography · MIC and CAI for Limited-resource Settings · Outcome Prediction

© The Author(s), under exclusive license to Springer Nature Switzerland AG 2025
R. Su et al. (Eds.): ISLES 2024/SWITCH 2024, LNCS 15408, pp. 3–11, 2025.
https://doi.org/10.1007/978-3-031-81101-2_1

# 1   Introduction

Intracerebral haemorrhage (ICH) accounts for a third of all strokes worldwide, but is responsible for a disproportionately high percentage of deaths, and ICH survivors often have severe disability. The Global Burden of Disease study showed that, between 1990 and 2010, 80% of ICH incidents were in low and middle income countries, where access to specialist stroke centres is limited [1]. ICH is caused by the rupture of a blood vessel in the brain, resulting in a large body of coagulating blood (haematoma) in the brain. This causes injury by mass effect; the compression and distortion of surrounding tissues due to increased pressure in the skull. The toxic byproducts of the breakdown of the haematoma can cause secondary injury to the surrounding tissue and swelling around the haematoma.

When a patient presents with stroke symptoms, they routinely receive a CT scan to identify the cause. If the stroke is caused by a clot, the patient can be treated immediately with clot dissolving medication or clot retrieval. If a bleed is identified, the rush is halted, as the only option for most patients is conservative management. Often, this diagnostic CT scan is the only form of imaging ICH patients will receive. There have been clinical trials of surgical haematoma evacuation, but whilst these trials have shown a modest reduction in mortality, no published studies have shown an improvement to functional outcome after ICH [2,3].

The corticospinal tract (CST) is a white matter tract that descends from the motor cortex through the midbrain and the brain stem, and is essential for fine motor and upper limb control. Damage to the CST from stroke results in poor motor recovery [4]. CST integrity can be assessed using imaging. The gold standard imaging method for white matter is diffusion tensor imaging (DTI), an MRI technique sensitive to the diffusion of water. Water diffuses with high anisotropy along white matter fibers, and low anisotropy in grey matter. The anisotropy and direction of diffusion can be measured by applying a direction sensitive gradient pulse. To build up a diffusion tensor, this gradient must be applied in at least 6 directions. From the diffusion tensor image, we can determine white matter streamlines, and map out the white matter tracts using probabilistic tractography.

DTI is often only used for ICH patients in a research setting, as it is not available in most centres due to cost, and is clinically challenging in acutely unwell patients. Unlike DTI, white/grey matter contrast on a CT scan is low. For ICH patients who only receive a diagnostic CT scan, assessing the integrity of the CST from CT is challenging.

Our aim was to develop a model that could produce tractography based labels of the CST from diagnostic CT scans alone. This tool would make white matter injury assessment available to all ICH patients with a diagnostic CT scan. This was done using paired CT and DTI scans of ICH patients to train a nnU-Net model [12] to delineate the CST on a CT scan. It was tested on a clinical trial dataset to investigate the clinical impact and utility of such a model and ask: can we use this automatic CT based assessment of CST integrity to predict motor outcome after stroke in the acute and chronic time frames? A CST assessment tool that only requires a CT scan could be used to probe clinical trial data for a subgroup of patients with intact CSTs, who may show a improvement in functional recovery after surgery. If successful, this could be used as a selection criteria for future clinical trials.

## 2   Methods

### 2.1   Data

The data used to develop the model for this study were taken from two clinical trials. The FETCH dataset is a multi-centre dataset of 152 ICH patients, 90 of whom were available to us, and received high-directional diffusion tensor imaging, T1, and CT imaging within a 5 day time frame [5]. The data were acquired at three different centres; Utrecht (n = 32, DTI acquired at 3T in 45 directions, Phillips), Leiden (n = 28, DTI acquired at 3T in 45 directions, Phillips) and Nijmegen (n = 32, DTI acquired at 3T in 64 directions, Siemens). The MISTIE III dataset was used to test the clinical utility of this model [2]. This is a clinical trial of surgical haematoma evacuation as an intervention for ICH. It consists of 499 patients randomised to either surgical intervention or medical treatment, all of whom received a diagnostic CT scan. The demographics of the MISTIE III clinical trial are shown in Table 1.

### 2.2   Diffusion Tensor Image Processing

To generate high quality tractography maps, several preprocessing steps were taken. Correction for susceptibility artefacts is usually done by using a b0 image acquired in the reverse phase encoding direction. The FETCH data, however, was only acquired in one phase encoding direction. To apply susceptibility correction, PreQual software, a deep learning based pipeline, was used to synthesise an artificial undistorted b0 image from a T1 image [6]. Synthesised b0 images were generated for the whole dataset, and PreQual was used to apply FSL's TopUp and Eddy Correction tools as per FSL's FDT pipeline.

FSL's Bayesian Estimation of Diffusion Parameters Obtained using Sampling Techniques Incorporating Crossing Fibres (BedpostX) was implemented on the corrected DTI data [7,8]. This technique is commonly used for mapping white matter tracts *in vivo* from whole brain diffusion imaging. BedpostX accounts for multiple fibres in different directions passing through any voxel by using the "ball-and-stick" model of diffusion [7,8]. The probability density functions of the diffusion parameters for each voxel are estimated using Markov Chain Monte Carlo sampling. A global streamline estimation can then be built by repeatedly sampling the probability density functions of the local diffusion parameters.

FSL's XTRACT tool was used to perform probabilistic tractography, and generate dissected white matter tract labels [9–11]. XTRACT is a wrapper for ProbtrackX, which samples the probability density functions produced by BedpostX, and adds anatomical seeds and stopping points. To allow tractography to be performed in each patient's native space, the anatomical seeds were registered from MNI to native space using EPI reg. The standard seed and stopping points for the CST are the peduncles and the motor cortex. For data from Leiden centre, anatomical seeds were selected several slices above the peduncles, due to obscuring artefacts in the midbrain.

The tractography maps were manually checked, and then linearly registered to native CT space using FSL FLIRT with a Correlation Ratio cost function. 80 tractography maps were successfully produced.

### 2.3   Model Training

We selected the self-adapting U-Net framework nnU-Net for our model architecture [12]. This is a framework that adapts the commonly used U-Net model according to the profile of the training data, and shows a vanilla U-Net can still perform at state of the art, if the parameters are carefully selected [13] .

A 3D full-resolution architecture was selected, consisting of a U-Net encoder-decoder structure. The encoder comprises six blocks, including the bottleneck, and the decoder five blocks. Each block includes two convolutional layers, each with a kernel size of $3 \times 3 \times 3$. The model was trained for 1000 epochs using a combination Dice and Cross Entropy loss on an NVIDIA a100 GPU, with a training dataset of 80 paired CT scans and CST labels (65 training, 15 testing). The data used for training and validation were selected using 5 fold cross-validation. The trained model was tested on the unseen testing dataset, and the testing ground truth and model predictions were compared using a Dice similarity coefficient.

To assess CST interaction with the haematoma, haematoma segmentations were manually drawn for 20 diagnostic CT scans from the MISTIE III dataset. A haematoma segmentation model was trained with these paired scans and labels (16 training, 4 testing) using the procedure outlined above.

### 2.4   Clinical Utility

To assess the clinical utility of such a model, we used the MISTIE III clinical trial dataset. Inference was run over 499 diagnostic ICH CT scans to generate predicted tractography masks of the CST and haematoma segmentations for each patient. From these CST and haematoma segmentations, measures of tract integrity were calculated. Two binary metrics of tract integrity were derived from the model predictions; haematoma overlap, and tract dissection. Haematoma overlap was defined to be true if the tractography segmentation overlapped with the haematoma segmentation in any voxel. Tract dissection was defined to be true if either side of the CST was not detected in any axial slice, implying an interruption or 'split' to the tract.

The MISTIE III dataset contains various stroke outcome data at different time points. In this work, we used the National Institute of Health Stroke Scale (NIHSS) score and the modified Rankin Scale (mRS) scale. The NIHSS score consists of a series of evaluations of a patient's neurological function, including consciousness, vision, motor function, coordination, and sensation. The score ranges from 0 to 42, with higher scores indicating more severe impairment. We used a sum of all scores in the motor domain, namely facial palsy, upper limbs (left and right), and lower limbs (left and right), to generate an overall 'motor' NIHSS score, ranging from 0–19. The mRS (modified Rankin Scale) is a measure used to assess the degree of disability or dependence in daily activities among patients who have suffered from a stroke or other neurological conditions. The scale ranges from 0–6, with 0 being no impairment, and 6 being death.

To investigate outcome in both the acute and chronic setting, we selected motor NIHSS at baseline (day 1), motor NIHSS at 180 d after stroke, and mRS at 365 d after stroke to be our outcome variables of interest.

Multiple linear regression analysis was conducted to assess the impact of CST integrity on our chosen outcome variables. We controlled for age, sex, natural logarithm of haematoma volume, intraventricular haemorrhage volume, and randomisation to surgical or medical treatment.

## 3   Results

Tractography maps were produced for 80 patients with DTI, T1 and CT imaging. Examples of the CST tractography maps for two patients can be seen in Fig. 1. Tractography failed for 10 patients.

The mean DSC between the ground truth tractography segmentations in the testing dataset and the CST model's predictions was 57%. Comparisons between the ground truth and model predictions for three patients can be seen in Fig. 2. The mean DSC between the ground truth haematoma segmentations in the testing dataset and the haematoma model's predictions was 94%.

Inference was run over diagnostic CT scans from the MISTIE III clinical trial dataset, and predicted labels of the CST and haematoma were generated for 487

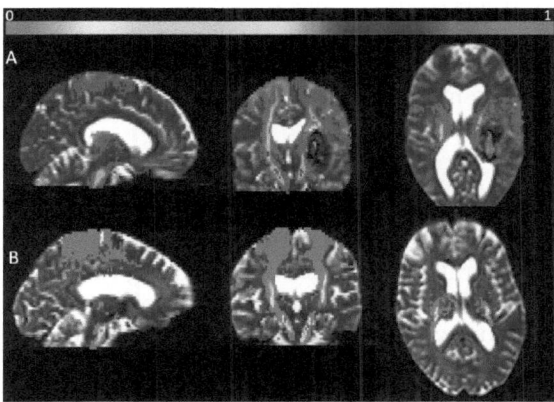

**Fig. 1.** Probabilistic tractography maps of the CST, superimposed onto the b0 volume of the DTI images for A) a patient with a haematoma involving the CST and B) a patient with a haematoma not involving the CST.

patients, three of whom are shown in Fig. 3. Demographics of the MISTIE III trial, split by CST integrity, are described in Table 1.

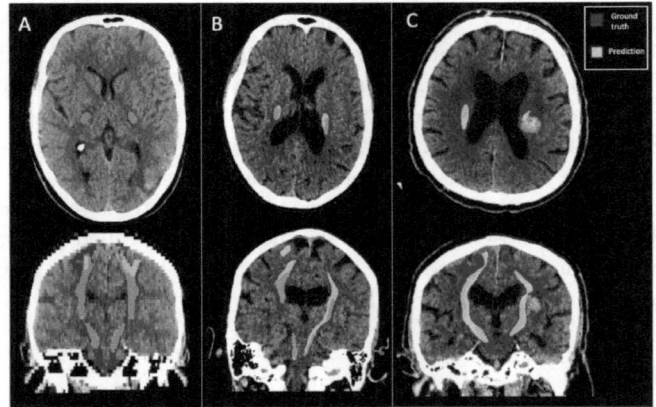

**Fig. 2.** Three test cases for the CST segmentation model. The ground truth DTI CST tractography is shown in purple, the model prediction is shown in cyan. A) A patient with a haematoma not involving the CST and a high DSC (DSC = 71%) B) A patient with a haematoma not involving the CST (DSC = 52%) C) A patient with a haematoma involving the CST (DSC = 66%).

Multiple linear regression analysis investigated the effect of haematoma overlap and tract dissection on the NIHSS stroke outcome metric. Both haematoma overlap and tract dissection were significantly associated with worse NIHSS score at baseline (p = 0.028, p < 0.0001 respectively) and at 180 d post stroke (p = 0.006, p < 0.0001 respectively). Tract dissection was associated with mRS at day 365 post stroke (p < 0.0001). Other significant predictors of outcome in the model were age, treatment group and natural logarithm of the haematoma volume. The results of the multiple linear regression analysis are shown in Table 2.

## 4 Discussion

DTI is the gold standard for white matter mapping, however, there are limitations to tractography in ICH patients. Fibre tracking can fail in close proximity to the haematoma and oedema, which are areas of low anisotropy. The mass effect of the haematoma can distort the surrounding anatomy, potentially rendering the seed points used in probabilistic tractography inaccurate. We see this in the 10 patients where tractography failed to produce reasonable white matter tracts. We also see this in the data from the Leiden centre, in which the tractography seed points had to be moved superiorly from the standard seed point in the peduncles, to avoid artefacts present in the midbrain. However, in

**Table 1.** Demographics of the MISTIE III clinical trial.

|  | All | CST involvement | No CST involvement | Tract split | No split |
|---|---|---|---|---|---|
|  | 487 | 110 | 377 | 170 | 317 |
| **Age** (mean) | 61.3 | 60.1 | 61.6 | 60.4 | 61.7 |
| **Sex** Male (n) | 299 | 81 | 218 | 113 | 186 |
| **Treatment group** |  |  |  |  |  |
| Surgery (n) | 247 | 59 | 188 | 89 | 158 |
| **Haematoma** |  |  |  |  |  |
| **volume** (mean) | 43.3 | 41.8 | 43.7 | 51.4 | 39.0 |
| **IVH** |  |  |  |  |  |
| **volume** (mean) | 2.4 | 2.5 | 2.4 | 3.8 | 1.6 |
| **NIHSS baseline** |  |  |  |  |  |
| (median [IQR]) | 10 [4] | 10 [4.5] | 10 [4] | 11 [4] | 9 [4] |
| **NIHSS day 180** |  |  |  |  |  |
| (median [IQR]) | 5 [7] | 6 [5] | 4 [6] | 6 [5] | 2 [6] |
| **mRS day 365** |  |  |  |  |  |
| (median [IQR]) | 4 [2] | 4 [2] | 4 [2] | 4 [2] | 3 [3] |

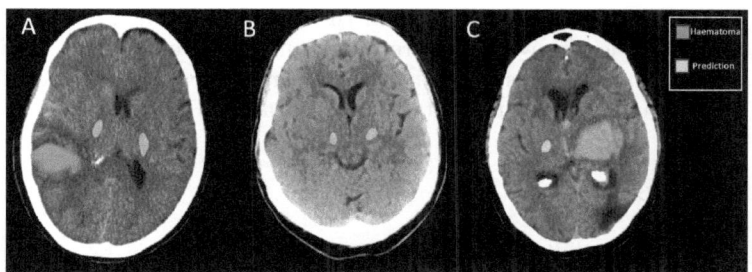

**Fig. 3.** Three patients from the MISTIE III dataset with predicted CST and haematoma labels. A) A patient with a haematoma not involving the CST B) A patient with CST haematoma overlap but no split tract C) A patient with no CST haematoma overlap, but a split tract.

**Table 2.** Multiple linear regression results.

|  |  | Haematoma overlap | Tract splitting |
|---|---|---|---|
| NIHSS day 1 | $\beta$ Coefficient [95% CI] | 0.94[0.10, 1.77] | 2.13 [1.38, 2.87] |
|  | p-value | 0.028* | <0.0001 **** |
| NIHSS day 180 | $\beta$ Coefficient [95% CI] | 1.32 [0.38, 2.25] | 3.55 [2.75, 4.36] |
|  | p-value | 0.006 ** | <0.0001 **** |
| mRS day 365 | $\beta$ Coefficient [95% CI] | 0.27 [-0.05, 0.58] | 0.86 [0.58, 1.14] |
|  | p-value | 0.097 (ns) | <0.0001 **** |

the 80 cases where tractography did not fail, reasonable maps of the CST were produced.

A DSC of 57% in the testing dataset is promising, as we are predicting the gold standard white matter imaging labels from a modality where the white/grey matter contrast is very low. A qualitative comparison of the models predictions in Fig. 2 shows an underestimation of the tract volume around the edges - this could be because the edges of the tract, where the fibre density is lower, are harder to see on a CT scan. The model is able to localise the CST in cases where there are gross changes to the brain structure, such as midline shift, suggesting it has not just learnt the relative distance from the tract to the skull.

We observe 'splits', interruptions in the z-axis, in the tract where the network cannot detect white matter. It is hard to say whether a split in the predicted tract is a reflection of damaged or undetectable white matter, or a failing of the model close to the haematoma. However, the fact that the presence of a 'split' very significantly predicts outcome after stroke shows that this does give us valuable information about CST integrity. It could be that combining discontinuity in the tract segmentation, and overlap with the haematoma would give us a comprehensive overview of whether a patient has damage to the CST.

In spite of the above limitations of tractography in ICH patients, and the low visibility of white matter in CT scans, the statistical results of the clinical trial analysis show that we have created a useful prognostic tool. This tool could be used in any centre with a CT scan in their stroke pipeline, enabling this to be used in the developing world, where the main burden of ICH lies. This could also be used for future investigations of whether surgical intervention for ICH leads to better outcomes for patients with an intact CST.

## 5    Conclusion

DTI based tractography is the gold standard for white matter delineation. However, most ICH patients will never receive a DTI scan, as it is both clinically challenging in acutely unwell patients, and unavailable in most diagnostic pipelines. We describe a nnU-Net based model that can predict tractography labels of the corticospinal tract from CT scans alone, with a dice similarity coefficient of 57%. We show that this model is clinically useful, and very significantly predicts outcome after stroke in the acute and chronic time frames in a large clinical trial. Our model, therefore, makes white matter injury assessment accessible to all patients who receive a diagnostic CT scan, allowing a prognosis of motor recovery from a diagnostic image for patients whom this information would be otherwise unavailable, and enabling future studies into targeted surgical interventions.

**Acknowledgments.** This study was funded through the MRC DTP iCASE studentship awarded to O.N. Murray

**Disclosure of Interests.** The authors have no competing interests

# References

1. An, S.J., Kim, T.J., Yoon, B.W.: Epidemiology, risk factors, and clinical features of intracerebral hemorrhage: an update. J. Stroke **19**(1), 3–10 (2017)
2. Hanley, D., Thompson, R., Rosenblum, M., et al.: Efficacy and safety of minimally invasive surgery with thrombolysis in intracerebral haemorrhageevacuation (MISTIE III): a randomised, controlled, open-label, blinded endpoint phase 3 trial. Lancet **393**(10175), 1021–1032 (2019)
3. Mendelow, A., Gregson, B., Rowan, E., et al.: Early surgery versus initial conservative treatment in patients with spontaneous supratentorial lobar intra cerebral haematomas (STICH II): a randomised trial. Lancet **382**(9890), 397–408 (2013)
4. Stinear, C., Barber, P., Smale, P., et al.: Functional potential in chronic stroke patients depends on corticospinal tract integrity. Brain: J. Neurol. **130**(Pt 1), 170–180 (2007)
5. Wiegertjes K, Voigt S, Jolink WMT, et al.: Diffusion-weighted lesions after intracerebral hemorrhage: associated MRI Findings. Front Neurol. **13**(882070), (2022)
6. Cai, L., Yang, Q., Hansen, C., et al.: PreQual: an automated pipeline for integrated preprocessing and quality assurance of diffusion weighted MRIimages. Magn. Reson. Med. **86**(1), 456–470 (2021)
7. Behrens, T., Woolrich, M., Jenkinson, M., et al.: Characterization and propagation of uncertainty in diffusion-weighted MR imaging. Magn. Reson. Med. **50**(5), 1077–1088 (2003)
8. Behrens T, Johansen-Berg H, Jbabdi S,et al.: Probabilistic diffusion tractography with multiple fibre orientations. What can we gain? NeuroImage **23**, 144–155 (2007)
9. Warrington S, Thompson E, Bastiani M, et al.: Concurrent mapping of brain ontogeny and phylogeny within a common space: standardized tractography and applications. Sci. Adv. **8**(42), (2022)
10. Warrington, S., Bryant, K., Khrapitchev, A., et al.: XTRACT - standardised protocols for automated tractography and connectivity blueprints in the human and macaque brain. NeuroImage **217**(116923) (2020)
11. de Groot, M., Vernooij, M.W., Klein, S., et al.: Improving alignment in Tract-based spatial statistics: evaluation and optimization of image registration. Neuroimage **76**(1), 400–411 (2013)
12. Isensee, F., Jaeger, P.F., Kohl, S.A., et al.: nnU-Net: a self-configuringmethod for deep learning-based biomedical image segmentation. Nat. Methods **18**(2), 203–211 (2021)
13. Isensee, F., Wald, T., Ulrich, C., et al.: nnU-Net revisited: a Call for rigorous validation in 3D medical image segmentation. arXiv:2404.09556 [cs.CV] (2024)

# Weakly Supervised Intracranial Hemorrhage Segmentation with YOLO and an Uncertainty Rectified Segment Anything Model

Pascal Spiegler[1]([✉]), Amirhossein Rasoulian[2], and Yiming Xiao[1]

[1] Department of Computer Science and Software Engineering, Concordia University, Montreal, Canada
pascal.spiegler@mail.concordia.ca
[2] NeuroRx Research, Montreal, Canada

**Abstract.** Intracranial hemorrhage (ICH) is a life-threatening condition that requires rapid and accurate diagnosis to improve treatment outcomes and patient survival rates. Recent advancements in supervised deep learning have greatly improved the analysis of medical images, but often rely on extensive datasets with high-quality annotations, which are costly, time-consuming, and require medical expertise to prepare. To mitigate the need for large amounts of expert-prepared segmentation data, we have developed a novel weakly supervised ICH segmentation method that utilizes the YOLO object detection model and an uncertainty-rectified Segment Anything Model (SAM). In addition, we have proposed a novel point prompt generator for this model to further improve segmentation results with YOLO-predicted bounding box prompts. Our approach achieved a high accuracy of 0.933 and an AUC of 0.796 in ICH detection, along with a mean Dice score of 0.629 for ICH segmentation, outperforming existing weakly supervised and popular supervised (UNet and Swin-UNETR) approaches. Overall, the proposed method provides a robust and accurate alternative to the more commonly used supervised techniques for ICH quantification without requiring refined segmentation ground truths during model training.

**Keywords:** Weak supervision · Image segmentation · Object detection · Medical imaging · Intracranial hemorrhage · YOLO · SAM

## 1 Introduction

Intracranial hemorrhage (ICH) accounts for 10–15% of all stroke cases and carries a significant risk of mortality [9]. Hemorrhage volume, which can rapidly expand within the first few hours, is a key predictor of treatment outcomes and potential complications [17]. Precise localization and quantification of the five ICH subtypes, including intraventricular (IVH), intraparenchymal (IPH), subarachnoid

R. Su et al. (Eds.): ISLES 2024/SWITCH 2024, LNCS 15408, pp. 12–21, 2025.
https://doi.org/10.1007/978-3-031-81101-2_2

(SAH), epidural (EDH), and subdural (SDH), are therefore essential for tailoring treatment strategies and minimizing adverse events [1]. While supervised deep learning (DL) models have demonstrated excellent potential in automating ICH assessment [7], their success heavily relies on large datasets with pixel-level annotations (ground-truth masks) and poor segmentation accuracy is observed with smaller training datasets [8]. However, large training datasets containing high-quality ground-truth masks are difficult to obtain due to high demands in time, labor, and domain expertise. Together with scarce public ICH segmentation datasets, this bottleneck poses great challenges in developing automatic ICH quantification algorithms to better facilitate the care and management of the condition.

To overcome the aforementioned issue, weakly supervised learning approaches [18,19] have emerged as a promising alternative. These methods leverage more economic ground truths, such as categorical labels, bounding boxes, or coarse masks to train segmentation models, bypassing the requirement of refined masks for fully supervised and semi-supervised approaches. While most existing literature is dedicated to ICH detection, ICH segmentation using weakly supervised methods remains under-explored. However, limited prior explorations exist leveraging explainable AI methods for weakly-supervised stroke segmentation, including class-activation maps (CAM) [25] and self-attention maps [19], providing encouraging results. Recent developments in foundation models, such as the Segment Anything Model (SAM) [10] have shown great potential to mitigate the segmentation ground truth bottleneck, but have not been explored for improving weakly supervised ICH segmentation. Therefore, we propose a novel weakly supervised ICH segmentation technique that incorporates automatic box and point prompt generation with SAM to allow for ICH detection and segmentation on CT scans. We have three main contributions. **First**, we leveraged a finetuned YOLOv8 model and a novel morphology-based method to automatically generate box and point prompts, respectively, for SAM. **Second**, to enhance segmentation accuracy with SAM, we employed an uncertainty rectification approach to account for uncertainty in prompt generation. **Lastly**, we explored the impacts of different prompt types for our proposed framework in ICH segmentation and compared it against state-of-the-art (SOTA) supervised and weakly supervised techniques.

## 2   Related Works

ICH segmentation methods still primarily rely on fully supervised approaches [2,3,11,12] and often with in-house datasets. More recently, semi-supervised techniques [24] have also been proposed for ICH quantification. However, refined segmentation ground truths are still crucial for their success, and more practical weakly supervised methods are gaining interest. In the limited prior works in this direction, most have relied on categorical labels as weak ground truths. For example, Wu et al. [25] proposed to use refined CAM results and representation learning to achieve ischemic stroke lesion segmentation, achieving a

0.3827 mean Dice score on multi-spectral MRIs. Later, from a binary classification CNN, Nemcek et al. [16] detected the location of ICH as bounding boxes in axial brain CT slices using the local extrema of derived attention maps, with a mean Dice of 0.58 for the lesion bounding boxes. Recently, Rasoulian et al. [19] utilized Head-Wise Gradient-Infused Self-Attention Maps from a Swin Transformer (Swin-HGI-SAM) trained on binary labels (ICH vs. no ICH) to obtain ICH segmentation, which obtained a mean Dice score of 0.438 on CT scans. The recent introduction of SAM [10], which allows interactive prompting in the forms of bounding boxes and/or points for zero-shot segmentation has attracted significant attention. However, its performance on CT-based ICH quantification and as an integrated solution allowing full automation in weakly supervised segmentation is yet to be explored. Furthermore, YOLO models [23] have been employed for ICH detection [4], but no reports have investigated their potential to facilitate the automation of SAM in ICH segmentation thus far.

## 3   Methods and Materials

### 3.1   Dataset and Preprocessing

For our study, we used the public Brain Hemorrhage Extended (BHX) dataset [20], which includes bounding box annotations for ICH along with their corresponding lesion subtypes, and the manually labeled PhysioNet CT dataset [8], which includes manual ICH segmentations. While 4607 CT slices and 5543 bounding boxes from the BHX dataset (containing the ICH subtypes and healthy scans) were employed to train and validate the YOLO model for lesion bounding box detection, the PhysioNet ICH segmentation dataset, which has 2814 CT slices with 318 mask-annotated ICH slices, was reserved as an independent test set to evaluate ICH segmentation with SAM. In addition, for our selected fully supervised baseline methods (more details in Sect. 3.3), subject-wise five-fold cross-validation was used on the manually segmented PhysioNet dataset to provide segmentation results for all cases and ensure that no slices from the same subject exist across different folds. As CT scans typically have a high dynamic range, for each CT slice, brain, subdural, and bone windows were created based on previous guidelines [5] and stacked together to form a composite RGB image, which was normalized to the range of [0,1] in each channel to facilitate training.

### 3.2   Uncertainty-Rectified YOLO-SAM Models

We propose YOLO-SAM, a novel weakly supervised framework for ICH segmentation, where the YOLOv8 model [23] provides several prompts for SAM to perform ICH segmentation. Here, we built three YOLO-SAM variants, including YOLO-SAM-BBox, YOLO-SAM-Point, and YOLO-SAM-PointBBox, which perform ICH segmentation using bounding box prompts, point prompts, and combinations of bounding boxes and point prompts, respectively. These models each employ an uncertainty rectification strategy that combines 10 SAM outputs

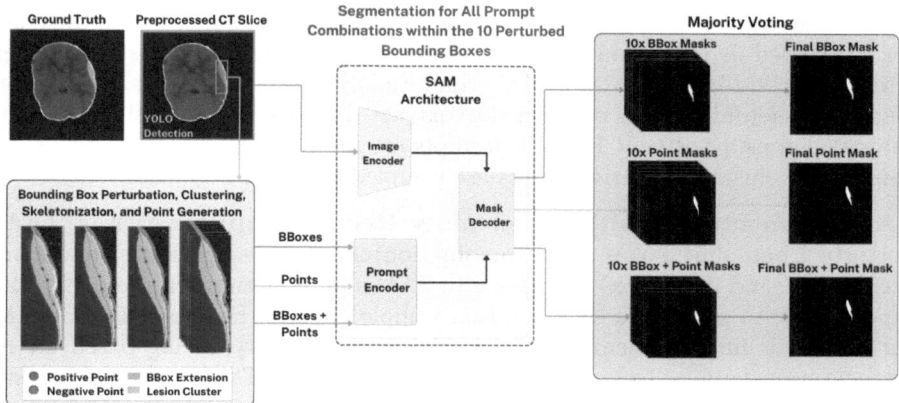

**Fig. 1.** Workflow of the proposed weakly supervised ICH segmentation method.

based on their 10 respective perturbed prompts. The detailed procedure of our methods is described below and shown in Fig. 1.

**YOLO Detection:** The preprocessed CT slices are passed to YOLOv8, which outputs the bounding boxes and associated lesion types for detected ICH. Then, the corner coordinates of the predicted bounding boxes are recorded to serve as the basis for automatic point prompt generation.

**Bounding Box Perturbations:** To enhance segmentation robustness and facilitate downstream uncertainty rectification in SAM's outputs, we introduce a method involving bounding box perturbation. Specifically, each YOLO-predicted bounding box is perturbed 10 times by randomly increasing its size by 1–4 pixels on each side. These perturbed boxes are recorded for the next step.

**Clustering and Point Prompt Generation:** Next, to strengthen the prompts' efficacy for SAM, leveraging the predicted ICH bounding box from YOLO, we introduce a novel point prompt generation method for the lesion and background based on a tailored tissue clustering solution and morphological analysis. To delineate lesions in proximity to the skull (e.g. SDH hemorrhage) for SAM, BET [22] skull-stripping is first applied to the entire CT image. Then, within the ICH bounding box for the skull-stripped RGB composite CT slice, K-means clustering is applied for tissue classification. Here, we use four clusters ($K = 4$) regardless of hemorrhage sub-types. If any residual skull is present, in decreasing order of the Hounsfield unit (HU) value, we must account for 1) residual skull tissue 2) ICH 3) healthy brain tissue and 4) dark background; if not, we can expect the brightest cluster to be assigned to the lesion and the remaining 3 clusters to be assigned to the rest. Then, an algorithm is devised to automatically identify the lesion cluster out of the four (YOLO-Clustering). The resulting simple tissue clustering is obtained by first inspecting whether the cluster with the highest average HU value corresponds to the brightest signals in the bone window channel, which represents the residual bone. If not, the cluster is selected as the lesion cluster. Otherwise, the algorithm picks the cluster with the second-highest average HU value. Finally, on the K-means-based lesion clusters, skeletonization is performed to extract the skeleton of the shapes. From these skeletons, positive ICH point prompts are sampled. Then, from each of the three other clusters, negative points are sampled for SAM segmentation.

**SAM Segmentation with Uncertainty Rectification:** For each of the 10 perturbed bounding boxes, each combination of generated prompts (bounding box, points, and point-box) are passed to SAM's prompt encoder along with the input image to produce a segmentation sample (Fig. 1). For each YOLO-SAM variant, their final segmentation is obtained via majority voting based on 10 segmentation samples from the associated prompt type. This voting mechanism ensures the robustness of ICH segmentation against network-related prompt instability and SAM's potential sensitivity to these variations, further improving segmentation quality.

### 3.3   Baseline Models and Ablation Study

To validate our proposed method, we compared its performance against the SOTA weakly supervised and fully supervised segmentation techniques for ICH segmentation. With an open-source repository and good performance, we chose the recent Swin-HGI-SAM [19] as our weakly supervised baseline. In terms of baseline methods with full supervision, we selected the popular UNet [21] and Swin-UNETR models [6], which have demonstrated strong performance in a wide range of medical image segmentation tasks. For the UNet model, we implemented the architecture from the manually segmented PhysioNet CT data paper [8], with four hierarchical layers in the encoding and decoding paths. For the Swin-UNETR model [6], we also adopted four hierarchical levels to be consistent with the UNet model.

While the SAM model [10] allows both bounding boxes and/or points as interactive prompts to generate segmentation results, the robustness and accuracy of individual prompt types and their combined usage still require further investigation. Therefore, besides comparison with the baseline models, we also performed an ablation study on the impact of prompt types for the target task (YOLO-SAM-Point, YOLO-SAM-BBox, YOLO-SAM-PointBBox).

### 3.4   Model Training and Evaluation Metrics

The YOLOv8-m model pretrained on the MS COCO dataset [13] in our YOLO-SAM variants was finetuned on the BHX dataset [20], with 3685 CT-slice images and 4479 bounding box labels for the training set, as well as 922 CT-slice images with 1064 labels for the validation set. We used the default YOLOv8 configuration (batch size=16, patience=100) during training. For the first 10,000 iterations, the AdamW optimizer was used with a learning rate of 0.00111 (calculated by a fitting equation using the number of bbox classes, which was 5 for each ICH subtype) and a momentum of 0.9. For the remaining iterations (after epoch 44), the SGD optimizer with an initial learning rate of 0.01 and momentum of 0.9 was used. We trained the weakly supervised Swin-HGI-SAM model [19] with the RSNA 2019 Brain CT hemorrhage dataset [5] (90%:10% data split for training vs. validation) following the details from the original publication. As for the supervised baselines (UNet and Swin-UNETR), subject-wise five-fold cross-validation was employed exclusively on the manually segmented PhysioNet dataset, using the AdamW optimizer with an initial learning rate of 0.001 as well as a loss function based on Dice coefficient and cross-entropy. We conducted all model training on a desktop computer with an Intel Core i9 CPU and an NVIDIA GeForce RTX 3090 GPU. *After model training, all evaluations were based on the manually segmented PhysioNet dataset in a slice-wise manner using the default YOLO confidence threshold of 0.25.* As ICH detection is a crucial component of our method, besides segmentation, we also evaluated the binary ICH detection performance (ICH vs. no ICH) for all DL models with accuracy, precision, recall, AUC, F1-score, and specificity. Note that a YOLO prediction was considered a true positive if it correctly identified a slice containing ICH, irrespective of the predicted subtype. For UNet and Swin-UNETR, a true-positive detection was defined as a slice with ICH segmentation that contains more than 10 pixels. In terms of segmentation, we computed the Dice coefficient and Intersection over Union (IoU) for all proposed and baseline models. Paired two-sample t-tests were then used to compare the Dice and IoU scores between the proposed method and the baselines, with $p < 0.05$ indicating a statistically significant difference.

## 4   Results

### 4.1   Detection Performance

**Table 1.** Detection Performance of Different Methods

| Metric | Swin-HGI-SAM | U-Net | Swin-UNETR | YOLOv8-m |
|---|---|---|---|---|
| Accuracy | 0.950 | 0.647 | 0.655 | 0.933 |
| Precision | 0.765 | 0.239 | 0.253 | 0.665 |
| Recall | 0.791 | 0.901 | 0.907 | 0.626 |
| AUC | 0.880 | 0.757 | 0.764 | 0.796 |
| F1-score | 0.767 | 0.373 | 0.374 | 0.645 |
| Specificity | 0.969 | 0.612 | 0.622 | 0.966 |

The ICH detection performance for all models is listed in Table 1. Similar to Swin-HGI-SAM, the YOLOv8-m model demonstrated superior detection performance for most metrics compared to the U-Net and Swin-UNETR models, particularly in precision (0.665 vs. 0.239 and 0.253), AUC (0.796 vs. 0.757 and 0.764), F1-score (0.645 vs. 0.373 and 0.374), and specificity (0.966 vs. 0.612 and

0.622). This highlights the potential of using bounding box localization models such as YOLO to achieve superior performance compared to mask-trained approaches on limited data (UNet, Swin-UNETR) and competitive performance with models trained on substantially more binary labels (Swin-HGI-SAM). However, a weakness of the YOLOv8-m model is its lower slice-wise recall compared to Swin-HGI-SAM (0.626 vs. 0.791), indicating that Swin-HGI-SAM will more reliably detect true positives. For all other detection metrics, YOLOv8-m demonstrated comparable but marginally weaker detection performance, likely due to the smaller number of training samples (4607 bounding box annotated CT slices for YOLO versus 677523 binary-labelled CT slices for Swin-HGI-SAM).

### 4.2   Segmentation Performance

The ICH segmentation results are shown in Table 2, with qualitative outcomes demonstrated in Fig. 2. Table 2 shows that point prompts, hybrid point and bounding box prompts, as well as simple tissue clustering within the YOLO bounding box (YOLO-Clustering) yielded significantly higher segmentation performance than Swin-HGI-SAM, UNet, Swin-UNETR and using bounding box prompts alone ($p < 0.005$). It is also shown that hybrid prompts have improved performance over point prompts and YOLO-Clustering on average, though not statistically significant ($p > 0.05$). While YOLO-Clustering had good segmentation quality, it also had higher standard error than SAM with hybrid and point prompts, highlighting the point prompt's better precision and reliability. Finally, while YOLO-SAM-BBox does not show significantly higher Dice and IoU scores than UNet ($p = 0.0853$) or Swin-UNETR ($p = 0.768$), it significantly outperforms Swin-HGI-SAM ($p < 0.005$).

**Table 2.** Segmentation Performance of Different Models (mean $\pm$ standard error)

| Model | Dice | IoU |
|---|---|---|
| Swin-HGI-SAM | $0.403 \pm 0.014$ | $0.283 \pm 0.011$ |
| Fully supervised U-Net | $0.388 \pm 0.019$ | $0.297 \pm 0.016$ |
| Fully supervised Swin-UNETR | $0.428 \pm 0.018$ | $0.330 \pm 0.011$ |
| YOLO-Clustering | $0.625 \pm 0.020$ | $0.506 \pm 0.019$ |
| YOLO-SAM-BBox | $0.562 \pm 0.020$ | $0.445 \pm 0.018$ |
| **YOLO-SAM-Point** | $\mathbf{0.627 \pm 0.018}$ | $\mathbf{0.506 \pm 0.017}$ |
| **YOLO-SAM-PointBBox** | $\mathbf{0.629 \pm 0.018}$ | $\mathbf{0.508 \pm 0.017}$ |

## 5   Discussion

Our YOLO-SAM framework that integrates YOLOv8-m, a novel point-prompt generator, and SAM with uncertainty rectification has demonstrated great performance in weakly supervised ICH segmentation, particularly with the hybrid

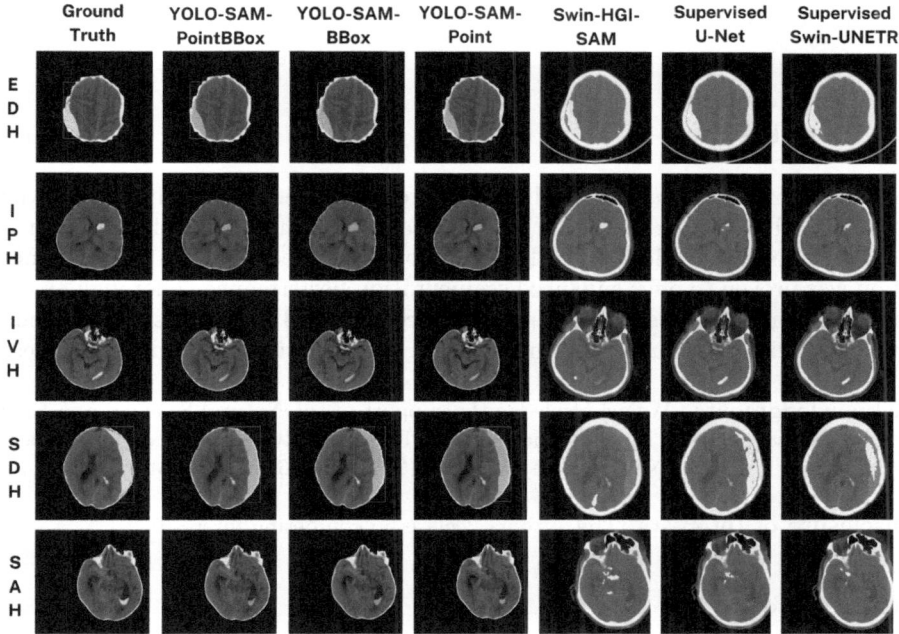

**Fig. 2.** Qualitative segmentation results on different ICH subtypes

prompts. The superior performance over existing weakly supervised and fully supervised methods can be explained by the incorporation of the power of the foundation models and spatial information represented by the bounding box ground truths. It is important to acknowledge that the poor performance of fully supervised DL models, such as UNet and Swin-UNETR can also be partially due to the low number of ground-truth mask labels. Despite this success, the slice-wise recall metric for our YOLO model lagged behind the Swin-HGI-SAM, suggesting a potential compromise in the model's ability to detect all ICH slices. However, after investigating this further on a patient-wise basis, the recall metric was calculated at 0.9714, with 34 out of 35 patients with hemorrhage having had at least one slice detected. In a clinical setting, the proportion of true positive ICH cases would therefore be much higher than the reported slice-wise recall metric. Our ablation study showed that hybrid prompts offered better performance than points or bounding boxes. This observation echoes previous reports [15] and could be explained by the lack of robustness when capturing thin, elongated, and curved structures (e.g., IPH subtype) with bounding boxes by SAM. Finally, while MedSAM [15] has gained great popularity in the community, its adoption in our YOLO-MedSAM-BBox model resulted in inferior segmentation outcomes (Dice = 0.412 ±0.018, IoU = 0.298 ±015). This is consistent with other reports of SAM outperforming MedSAM on certain medical image segmentation tasks [14] and may be due to a lack of public datasets for training MedSAM on ICH tasks, as Dice loss was used in training the model [15].

## 6   Conclusion

In conclusion, we have proposed a novel weakly supervised ICH segmentation technique that uses YOLO and an uncertainty-rectified SAM. In addition to bounding boxes provided via YOLO, our morphology-based point prompt generation was proven to offer enhanced segmentation performance. Thorough assessments have revealed its superior performance over SOTA weakly supervised and fully supervised baselines while maintaining strong ICH detection capabilities.

**Acknowledgments.** We acknowledge the support of the Natural Sciences and Engineering Research Council of Canada (596537, RGPIN/05100-2022) and the Fonds de recherche du Québec - Nature et technologies (2022-PR296459, B1X-348625).

**Disclosure of Interests.** The authors declare no competing interests.

## References

1. Aguilar, M.I., Brott, T.G.: Update in intracerebral hemorrhage. Neurohospitalist **1**(3), 148–159 (2011)
2. Chang, P.D., et al.: Hybrid 3d/2d convolutional neural network for hemorrhage evaluation on head ct. Am. J. Neuroradiol. **39**(9), 1609–1616 (2018)
3. Cho, J., et al.: Improving sensitivity on identification and delineation of intracranial hemorrhage lesion using cascaded deep learning models. J. Digit. Imaging **32**, 450–461 (2019)
4. Ertuğrul, Ö.F., Akıl, M.F.: Detecting hemorrhage types and bounding box of hemorrhage by deep learning. Biomed. Signal Process. Control **71**, 103085 (2022)
5. Flanders, A.E., et al.: Construction of a machine learning dataset through collaboration: the rsna 2019 brain ct hemorrhage challenge. Radiology: Artifi. Intell. **2**(3), e190211 (2020)
6. Hatamizadeh, A., Nath, V., Tang, Y., Yang, D., Roth, H.R., Xu, D.: Swin unetr: swin transformers for semantic segmentation of brain tumors in mri images. In: International MICCAI Brainlesion Workshop, pp. 272–284. Springer (2021). https://doi.org/10.1007/978-3-031-08999-2_22
7. Heit, J., et al.: Automated cerebral hemorrhage detection using rapid. Am. J. Neuroradiol. **42**(2), 273–278 (2021)
8. Hssayeni, M.D., Croock, M.S., Salman, A.D., Al-khafaji, H.F., Yahya, Z.A., Ghoraani, B.: Intracranial hemorrhage segmentation using a deep convolutional model. Data **5**(1) (2020)
9. Isabel C. Hostettler, D.J.S., Werring, D.J.: Intracerebral hemorrhage: an update on diagnosis and treatment. Expert Rev. Neurotherapeutics **19**(7), 679–694 (2019), pMID: 31188036
10. Kirillov, A., et al.: Segment anything. In: Proceedings of the IEEE/CVF International Conference on Computer Vision, pp. 4015–4026 (2023)

11. Kuo, W., Häne, C., Yuh, E., Mukherjee, P., Malik, J.: Cost-sensitive active learning for intracranial hemorrhage detection. In: Frangi, A.F., Schnabel, J.A., Davatzikos, C., Alberola-López, C., Fichtinger, G. (eds.) MICCAI 2018. LNCS, vol. 11072, pp. 715–723. Springer, Cham (2018). https://doi.org/10.1007/978-3-030-00931-1_82
12. Lee, H., et al.: An explainable deep-learning algorithm for the detection of acute intracranial haemorrhage from small datasets. Nat. Biomed. Eng. **3**(3), 173–182 (2019)
13. Lin, T.-Y., et al.: Microsoft COCO: common objects in context. In: Fleet, D., Pajdla, T., Schiele, B., Tuytelaars, T. (eds.) ECCV 2014. LNCS, vol. 8693, pp. 740–755. Springer, Cham (2014). https://doi.org/10.1007/978-3-319-10602-1_48
14. Liu, H., Yang, H., van Diest, P.J., Pluim, J.P., Veta, M.: Wsi-sam: multiresolution segment anything model (sam) for histopathology whole-slide images. arXiv preprint arXiv:2403.09257 (2024)
15. Ma, J., He, Y., Li, F., Han, L., You, C., Wang, B.: Segment anything in medical images. Nat. Commun. **15**(1), 654 (2024)
16. Nemcek, J., Vicar, T., Jakubicek, R.: Weakly supervised deep learning-based intracranial hemorrhage localization. arXiv preprint arXiv:2105.00781 (2021)
17. Qureshi, A., Palesch, Y.: Antihypertensive treatment of acute cerebral hemorrhage (atach) ii: design, methods, and rationale. Neurocrit. Care **15**, 559–576 (2011)
18. Rasoulian, A., Salari, S., Xiao, Y.: Weakly supervised intracranial hemorrhage segmentation using hierarchical combination of attention maps from a swin transformer. In: Machine Learning in Clinical Neuroimaging, pp. 63–72. Springer Nature Switzerland, Cham (2022). https://doi.org/10.1007/978-3-031-17899-3_7
19. Rasoulian, A., Salari, S., Xiao, Y.: Weakly Supervised Intracranial Hemorrhage Segmentation using Head-Wise Gradient-Infused Self-Attention Maps from a Swin Transformer in Categorical Learning. arXiv (Cornell University) (Jan 2023)
20. Reis, E., et al.: Brain hemorrhage extended (bhx): bounding box extrapolation from thick to thin slice ct images (July 2020)
21. Ronneberger, O., Fischer, P., Brox, T.: U-Net: convolutional networks for biomedical image segmentation. In: Navab, N., Hornegger, J., Wells, W.M., Frangi, A.F. (eds.) MICCAI 2015. LNCS, vol. 9351, pp. 234–241. Springer, Cham (2015). https://doi.org/10.1007/978-3-319-24574-4_28
22. Smith, S.M.: Fast robust automated brain extraction. Hum. Brain Mapp. **17**(3), 143–155 (2002)
23. Terven, J., Córdova-Esparza, D.M., Romero-González, J.A.: A comprehensive review of yolo architectures in computer vision: from yolov1 to yolov8 and yolo-nas. Mach. Learn. Knowl. Extract. **5**(4), 1680–1716 (2023)
24. Wang, J.L., Farooq, H., Zhuang, H., Ibrahim, A.K.: Segmentation of intracranial hemorrhage using semi-supervised multi-task attention-based u-net. Appl. Sci. **10**(9), 3297 (2020)
25. Wu, K., Du, B., Luo, M., Wen, H., Shen, Y., Feng, J.: Weakly supervised brain lesion segmentation via attentional representation learning. In: Shen, D., et al (eds.) MICCAI 2019. LNCS, vol. 11766, pp. 211–219. Springer, Cham (2019). https://doi.org/10.1007/978-3-030-32248-9_24

# Bayesian Uncertainty Estimation Improves nnU-Net Generalization to Unseen Sites for Stroke Lesion Segmentation

Linda Vorberg[1,2](✉)(ID), Hendrik Ditt[2](ID), Michael Sühling[2](ID), Andreas Maier[1](ID), Nicolas Murray[3](ID), Savvas Nicolaou[3](ID), and Oliver Taubmann[2](ID)

[1] Friedrich-Alexander-Universität Erlangen-Nürnberg, Erlangen, Germany
`linda.vorberg@fau.de`
[2] CT R&D Image Analytics, Siemens Healthineers, Forchheim, Germany
[3] Department of Radiology, Vancouver General Hospital, University of British Columbia, Vancouver, Canada

**Abstract.** This work studies the effectiveness of Bayesian uncertainty estimation in neural networks for enhancing domain generalization in stroke lesion segmentation. We employ a multi-modal posterior sampling approach for nnU-Net and evaluate it against the conventional nnU-Net. Both models are trained on data from one clinical site and tested on another for the most common imaging in stroke: NCCT, CTA, and CTP. The models produce segmentation probabilities for stroke core and hypoperfused tissue, which are thresholded at different levels and compared to ground truth labels to measure correctly predicted, missing and excess volume, and Dice scores. Conventional nnU-Net is limited in sensitivity adjustment, while the Bayesian approach allows for a flexible trade-off between under- and over-segmentation. The Bayesian nnU-Net demonstrates similar or superior performance w.r.t. Dice scores, with the added advantage of providing more insight into uncertain areas, enabling more nuanced decision-making. The Bayesian approach proved robust in handling data from unseen domains, suggesting its potential for enhancing automated stroke lesion detection across various clinical environments.

**Keywords:** Stroke Segmentation · Uncertainty Estimation · Domain Generalization

## 1 Introduction

Stroke is a severe medical condition characterized by a sudden loss of brain function, which is caused by a lack of blood supply from a blocked vessel in the ischemic case [8]. Timely and accurate diagnosis is crucial for the patient's outcome and requires the use of medical imaging tools and their assessment. In the field of automated image analysis, especially segmentation of, e.g. stroke lesions, Deep Learning (DL)-based models have come into play [1]. Extensive

R. Su et al. (Eds.): ISLES 2024/SWITCH 2024, LNCS 15408, pp. 22–30, 2025.
https://doi.org/10.1007/978-3-031-81101-2_3

research has been performed in stroke lesion segmentation and identification with neural networks, involving all relevant kinds of CT images types, namely Non-Contrast CT (NCCT), CT Angiography (CTA), CT Perfusion (CTP) [4,6,10]. A major drawback of most neural networks trained for diagnosis support is the lack of generalization on unseen data. Networks tend to be overconfident on data that stems from a different domain, including different clinical sites, imaging protocols, scanning parameters and configurations, and patient demographics. DL models have been shown to output confident predictions when confronted with out-of-distribution data, which can be considered poor calibration of the model [2,5]. This overconfidence can lead to erroneous clinical decisions, as the probabilities output by these networks often do not reflect true uncertainties.

To address this challenge, uncertainty-aware deep learning models have been proposed. These models aim to provide more accurate probability estimates by incorporating mechanisms to quantify uncertainty. Techniques such as Bayesian neural networks and ensemble methods have shown promise in calibrating the confidence of DL models, thereby improving their reliability and robustness in clinical practice [12]. This work explores the use of a Bayesian uncertainty estimation technique for the nnU-Net framework [3,11] and tests its abilities for the generalization to an unseen site. To this end, we employ models to segment stroke core and surrounding penumbra on all common CT scans – NCCT, CTA and CTP –, training on data from one clinical site and testing on another. The performance on this task is compared between the conventional nnU-Net and the Bayesian approach to investigate the capabilities of domain adaptation.

## 2    Materials and Methods

### 2.1    Dataset

Two datasets are used in this study to investigate the aspect of site transfer. The first dataset (Center A) was acquired with a Somatom Definition AS+ scanner (Siemens Healthineers, Forchheim, Germany) at the Universitätsklinikum Schleswig-Holstein, Lübeck, and comprises NCCT, CTA and CTP scans of 166 patients. The mean infarct core size in this patient cohort was $34.5 \pm 37.3$ ml. Stroke onset times, which are particularly relevant regarding the visibility of ischemic changes on NCCT scans, were not available. The average resolution of the three different CT image types is $0.43 \times 0.43 \times 0.8 \, \text{mm}^3$, $0.64 \times 0.64 \times 0.53 \, \text{mm}^3$ and $0.43 \times 0.43 \times 1.0 \, \text{mm}^3$. NCCT scans were acquired with tube voltages of 100 to 140 kV, CTA with 80 to 120 kV and CTP with 80 kV. The second dataset comes from Vancouver General Hospital, Canada (Center B) and includes 95 patients that were all examined using a Somatom Force (Siemens Healthineers, Forchheim, Germany) Dual Energy CT (DECT) scanner. Here, the NCCT and CTA scans are acquired using two different energy levels, 90 and 150 kV, and CTP with a tube voltage of 70 kV. NCCT, CTA and CTP scans are available with an average resolution of $0.45 \times 0.45 \times 0.99 \, \text{mm}^3$, $0.50 \times 0.50 \times 0.70 \, \text{mm}^3$ and $0.41 \times 0.41 \times 2.98 \, \text{mm}^3$. 89 patients showed with an acute ischemic infarct (mean volume: $13.3 \pm 18.1$), while the remaining 6 patients only showed a prior infarction. For both datasets, all available cases were included in the experiments. For annotation purposes, CT perfusion maps derived from the CTP scans, showing Cerebral Blood Volume (CBV), Cerebral Blood Flow (CBF) and Time to Maximum Enhancement (TMAX), were used.

## 2.2   Labels

Reference annotations for the datasets are performed based on the labeling scheme described by Vorberg et al. [9]. For both ischemic core and hypoperfused volume, which is the composite of core and surrounding penumbra, a minimum and maximum boundary is delineated assessing perfusion deficits on CBV, CBF and TMAX and omitting artifacts, e.g. those at the base of the skull. These boundaries capture the uncertainty inherent to the task of contouring these two classes on perfusion maps. The area within the inner boundary marks the minimum extent of the class, while the outer boundary captures its maximum extent beyond which no occurrence of the specific tissue is assumed. As this work intends to assess generalizability and uncertainty estimation directly using a Bayesian approach, a single contour is derived for training of both classes. For this purpose, the area between the inner and outer boundary is transformed into a relative distance map based on the Euclidean distance transform. This distance map is then thresholded at 0.5 to obtain a single contour, which reflects the extent of the tissue that lies exactly between inner and outer boundary. In addition to the core and hypoperfused volume label, the network is presented with a third label delineating prior infarcts such that it learns to distinguish those from acute infarctions.

## 2.3   Bayesian nnU-Net Sampling

To explore a neural network for image segmentation that directly captures uncertainty, a Bayesian variant of the well-known nnU-Net [3] was used in this study, following the approach described in [11]. The authors propose a posterior sampling of the weight space to estimate uncertainty. By choosing the "Multi Modal Posterior Sampling" method, the problem of converging in a local optimum and therefore only capturing one mode of the weight posterior is overcome through a cyclical learning rate scheme. Hereby, the total number of epochs $T$ is divided into $M$ cycles, where the learning rate is initially high for the first epoch of the cycle ($\alpha_r$). Then, it decays until a fixed fraction ($\gamma$) of the epochs in the cycle is reached and the learning rate is kept constant. This is described by the formula,

$$\alpha(t) = \begin{cases} \alpha_r & \text{if } t_c = 0 \\ \alpha_0 \left[1 - \frac{\min(t_c, \gamma T_c)}{T}\right]^{\epsilon} & \text{if } t_c > 0 \end{cases} \tag{1}$$

with $T_c = T/M$ and $t_c = t \mod T_c$ with $t$ being the current epoch. $\epsilon$ controls the decay of the learning rate $\alpha$. The weight sampling is performed at the end of each cycle c, collecting checkpoints $\boldsymbol{W}_c = \{\boldsymbol{w}_t \mid \gamma T_c \leq t \mod T_c \leq T_c - 1\}$ within the epochs where the learning rate is kept constant and the learning has stabilized. Doing this for all $M$ cycles builds an ensemble of $n \cdot M$ models with intermediate weights from each mode. In this way, both the local and global uncertainty in the weights is captured. At inference time, the samples of the test set are passed into all individual models and their predictions are averaged.

### 2.4    Experimental Setup

**Input Data.** The models are all trained on the data from Center A and tested on the unseen domain, the data from center B. As input into the Bayesian as well as the baseline network, NCCT, CTA and CTP images were used. CTP scans consist of multiple 3D volumes, acquired at subsequent time points (here between 28 and 44). To utilize these scans for network training, the temporal dimension was reduced by selecting three specific time points $t_i, i \in \{0, 1, 2\}$ from the series, averaging a window of three subsequent scans around each $t_i$. In this study, the timing of these windows was chosen similar to the timing in a multi-phase CTA protocol and is facilitated by the time-attenuation curve (TAC) of the arterial input function that is obtained by a perfusion evaluation algorithm. The first time point $t_0$ is set two time points before the arterial peak of the TAC. $t_1$ and $t_2$ follow 13 s and 21 s after the initial phase, respectively. This results in three phases of the CTP scan that are concatenated as channels forming the input into the network. All images are registered and resampled to the motion correction baseline time point of the CTP scan. For the CTP scans of Center A, that originally have a slice thickness of 1 mm, thicker slices of 5 mm were synthesized to reduce noise.

**Uncertainty Experiments.** nnU-Net was trained with the Multi-Modal checkpoint sampling method on the data from Center A. Individual models were trained for each type of CT scan, NCCT, CTA and CTP, with all of the patients available. The parameters for the learning rate scheduling were defined as in [11]. 1200 epochs ($T$) were trained, split up into $M = 3$ cycles with $\alpha_r = 0.1$, $\alpha_0 = 0.01$ and $\epsilon = 0.9$. The learning rate was kept constant after $\gamma = 0.8$ of the epochs in each cycle. The last ten epochs per cycle were sampled, resulting in a total of 30 checkpoints that were used for inference.

**Baseline Experiments.** To compare against conventional nnU-Net training without uncertainty estimation, the framework was used in its standard setting, also training three individual models on all of the available patients from Center A. At test time, inference was done with the data from Center B, predicting stroke core and hypoperfused volume based on the final checkpoint of the model. Additionally, the probability values of the network output were stored for later analysis.

## 2.5   Evaluation

**Threshold Sweep.** After testing the images from the test set on all model checkpoints obtained during the training of the Bayesian nnU-Net, the discrete predictions for each label are averaged, forming a probability map for every label predicted, as shown in the 4th row of Fig. 2. Applying a threshold to this probabilistic prediction implies the selection of a level of certainty, as this determines the extent of the predicted tissue, e.g. stroke core. To investigate this effect, a threshold sweep is performed, similar to what is done in ROC analysis, comparing different thresholds with the model's segmentation performance. The same can be done for the output of the normal nnU-Net model, as the network also produces "probabilities" (2nd row of Fig. 2) that are usually thresholded at 0.5 to obtain a single prediction.

**Metrics.** For evaluation purposes, a modified Dice score as well as volumetric measures are assessed. As the original labels include a delineation of minimum and maximum extent of core and hypoperfused area, the prediction is compared to both the inner and outer contour of the tissue of interest delivering a more fine-grained analysis of the predicted areas. Using this approach, areas within the inner label that are not part of the predicted volume are counted as missing volume and predicted areas outside of the outer label are denoted excess volume. Consequently, predicted areas enclosed by the outer contour are correctly predicted. Based on this concept, the original formulation of the Dice score is modified to,

$$D(A, B_I, B_O) = \frac{2 \cdot |A \cap B_O|}{|A| + |B_I| + |A \cap (B_O \setminus B_I)|}. \tag{2}$$

with the prediction $A$, and $B_I$ and $B_O$ describing the regions enclosed by the inner and outer boundary of the ground truth label, respectively.

## 3   Results

The effect of the threshold applied to the prediction of the models on the performance is shown in Fig. 1. The probability output of nnU-Net is the output of the softmax function at the end of the network. An example is encoded in the heatmap in the second row of Fig. 2. For the Bayesian variant, the probability maps stem from the averaged discrete predictions for each label that result from the model checkpoints sampled during training. An example is shown in the 4th row of Fig. 2. Figure 1a displays the threshold sweep for the normal nnU-Net, where it can be observed that the modified Dice is quite stable across the thresholds. Only on the lower and upper end of the threshold range, the modified Dice value is rapidly declining, as e.g. at a threshold below 0.01, the whole image would be segmented and classified into one class, which results into a very high excess volume and a loss of specificity. Varying the threshold applied to the averaged predictions of the Bayesian nnU-Net yields the curves plotted in Fig. 1b.

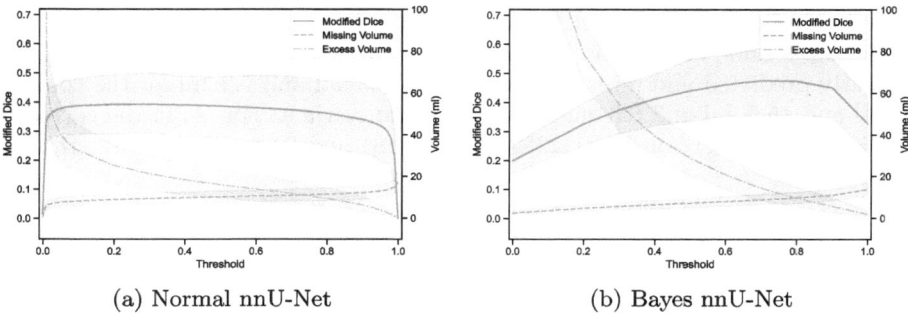

(a) Normal nnU-Net                          (b) Bayes nnU-Net

**Fig. 1.** Modified Dice, missing and excess volume with 95% confidence intervals plotted against the thresholds applied to the probability output. 1a shows the result for the conventional nnU-Net, 1b for the Bayesian approach. Both experiments were performed with NCCT scans in the subgroup of 10–70 ml infarcts.

**Table 1.** Modified Dice values (mean ± std) for the prediction of stroke core. The best threshold is assessed on the nnU-Net heatmap (conventional nnU-Net) or the checkpoint-ensembled probability map (Bayes nnU-Net). All models are trained on the data from Center A and tested on Center B.

| Model | Data | Best Threshold | Volume Group $1 < x < 10$ ml | Volume Group $10 < x < 70$ ml | Volume Group $x > 70$ ml |
|---|---|---|---|---|---|
| nnU-Net | NCCT | 0.1 | $0.11 \pm 0.16$ | $0.38 \pm 0.23$ | $\mathbf{0.68 \pm 0.28}$ |
| Bayes nnU-Net | NCCT | 0.7 | $\mathbf{0.14 \pm 0.18}$ | $\mathbf{0.46 \pm 0.26}$ | $0.65 \pm 0.27$ |
| nnU-Net | CTA | 0.1 | $0.20 \pm 0.26$ | $0.56 \pm 0.23$ | $0.56 \pm 0.40$ |
| Bayes nnU-Net | CTA | 0.6 | $\mathbf{0.24 \pm 0.24}$ | $\mathbf{0.59 \pm 0.20}$ | $\mathbf{0.65 \pm 0.37}$ |
| nnU-Net | CTP | 0.1 | $0.45 \pm 0.30$ | $\mathbf{0.80 \pm 0.09}$ | $0.80 \pm 0.19$ |
| Bayes nnU-Net | CTP | 0.5 | $\mathbf{0.47 \pm 0.30}$ | $\mathbf{0.80 \pm 0.09}$ | $\mathbf{0.81 \pm 0.15}$ |

Here, the modified Dice shows a larger variation with the application of different thresholds and a higher maximum than for the conventional nnU-Net.

The modified Dice scores for the experiments involving the various scans are shown across different volume groups in Table 1. These subgroups are defined based on the ground truth core volume and result in 46, 24, and 2 cases in the groups $1 < x < 10$ ml, $10 < x < 70$ ml and $x > 70$ ml respectively, discarding 23 cases with $x < 1$ ml, as done in [7], where these cases are regarded irrelevant. Results are given for the threshold yielding the highest metric, assessed on the whole dataset. For all scans, using the Bayesian approach exhibits better modified Dice scores than the conventional nnU-Net across all subgroups, except for the largest volume group (with only 2 cases) when using NCCT images. Generally, the more involved scans with admission of contrast agent, CTA and CTP, achieve a higher performance than the NCCT scans, with the highest Dice score of 0.8 achieved with CTP in middle sized infarcts. In this case, the performance of the conventional nnU-Net is on par with the Bayesian approach. In addition to the modified Dice scores, volumetric measurements were assessed comparing the prediction to the ground truth label. For NCCT images, the mean correctly predicted volume is 14.4 ml for the conventional nnU-Net and 12.3 ml for the

Bayesian approach for infarcts of size 10–70 ml (mean volume 23.9 ml), with a missing volume of 7.5 ml (8.3 ml). Regarding the same subgroup for CTA, correctly predicted and missing volumes are 13.3 ml and 7.5 ml for the conventional and 15.5 ml and 6.3 ml for the Bayesian variant. For CTP, the correctly predicted (missing) volume is 22.4 ml (2.2 ml) and 21.4 ml (2.5 ml), respectively.

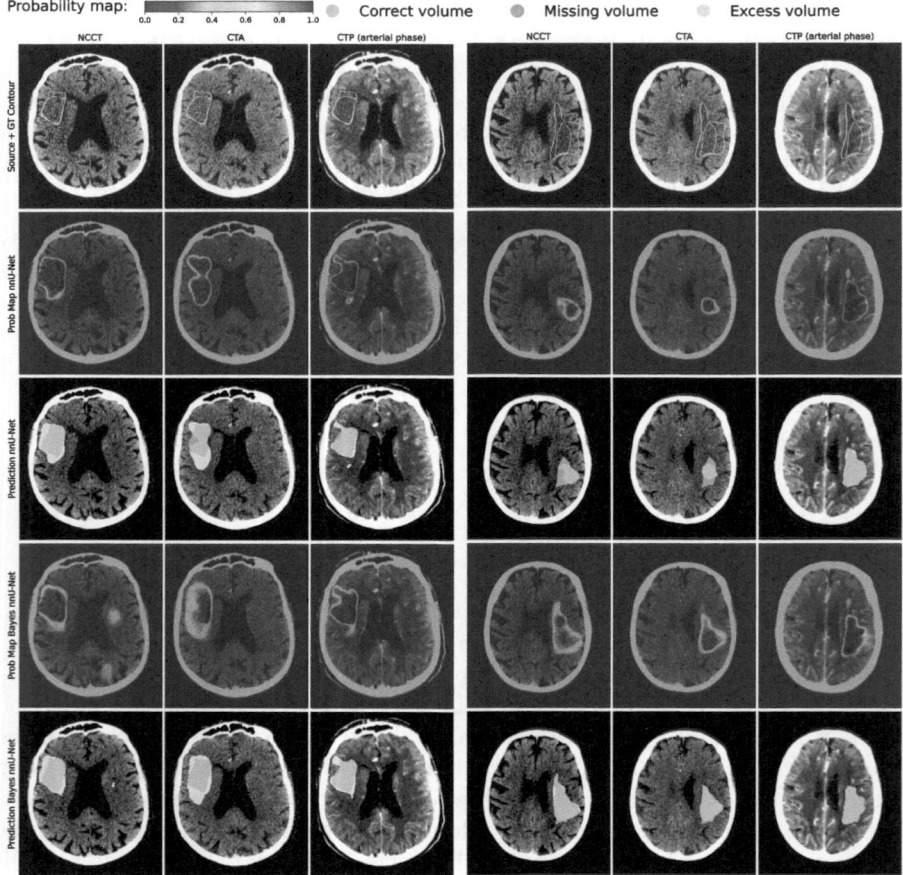

**Fig. 2.** Two example cases: 1st row shows a slice of the respective scan with the ground truth inner and outer contour of stroke core. The 2nd and 4th row show the probability maps of the conventional and the Bayesian nnU-Net. The predicted probabilities of each model are thresholded at 0.5 and compared against the ground truth (3rd and 5th row).

## 4    Discussion and Conclusion

We investigate the use of uncertainty estimation in neural networks for generalization to unseen sites in stroke lesion segmentation. A Bayesian variant for the nnU-Net framework is employed, using a multi modal posterior sampling approach that captures local and global uncertainty. To asses the generalization capabilities of this network, it is compared to a standard nnU-Net. Both models are trained on data from one clinical site and tested on another, using different scans involved in stroke diagnosis, namely NCCT, CTA and CTP. The networks yield output probabilities for the segmentation labels for stroke core and hypoperfused tissue that can be thresholded at different levels. The resulting label is compared against ground truth inner and outer contours of the tissue of interest to assess correct, missing and excess predicted volume and modified Dice scores.

The analysis of the threshold sweep shows that the predicted probabilities of the conventional nnU-Net are often nearly binary, offering limited sensitivity/specificity adaptation. Although the Bayesian approach also shows limitations in performance, particularly with NCCT scans, it allows for a variable trade-off between under- and over-segmentation by applying appropriate thresholds. Overall, the Bayesian nnU-Net outperforms its conventional counterpart across all scan types in (nearly) all volume groups regarding the modified Dice scores. The benefit is slightly lower when using CTP scans, where both networks achieve a modified Dice of 0.8 and similar volumetric measures for middle sized infarcts, likely due to the contrast enhancement and temporal information present in these scans which makes lesions easier to delineate. This is also reflected in the heatmap of the network output in the $4^{th}$ row of Fig. 2, where the probabilities vary less for the perfusion scan, indicating higher certainty. While determining the ideal threshold for binary segmentation on the unseen domain may require (a small number of) tuning data sets in practice, the results demonstrate that only the Bayesian approach stands to gain significantly from it.

Inspecting the example cases and their network output in Fig. 2 highlights its primary advantage beyond performance gains in modified Dice scores. Areas of uncertainty are mostly present in the probability output of the Bayesian network ($4^{th}$ row), but only barely in the ones from the conventional nnU-Net ($2^{nd}$ row). The relatively stable performance over different thresholds demonstrates robustness but such overconfident predictions can be problematic when running inference on data from an unseen site. In contrast, the Bayesian network offers flexibility and insights into areas of uncertainty, providing valuable information for decision-making and allowing to visualize the full range of likely lesion extents. For instance, in the case shown on the right-hand side of Fig. 2, the infarct core appears severely underestimated by the conventional nnU-Net on NCCT and CTA regardless of the threshold applied whereas the Bayesian distribution covers the annotation well and yields an accurate segmentation with the default threshold of 0.5.

In conclusion, the use of a Bayesian sampling approach to DL-based models can be a valuable tool for clinicians to better understand and manage inherent uncertainties in medical imaging, potentially enhancing the reliability and applicability of automated stroke lesion detection across different clinical sites.

**Acknowledgments.** We sincerely thank our collaborators from Universitätsklinikum Schleswig-Holstein Lübeck, Germany, for providing the data used in this study.

# References

1. Cui, L., et al.: Deep learning in ischemic stroke imaging analysis: a comprehensive review. Biomed. Res. Int. **2022**(1), 2456550 (2022)
2. Guo, C., Pleiss, G., Sun, Y., Weinberger, K.Q.: On calibration of modern neural networks. In: International Conference on Machine Learning, pp. 1321–1330. PMLR (2017)
3. Isensee, F., Jaeger, P.F., Kohl, S.A., Petersen, J., Maier-Hein, K.H.: nnU-Net: a self-configuring method for deep learning-based biomedical image segmentation. Nat. Methods **18**(2), 203–211 (2021)
4. Lin, S.Y., et al.: Toward automated segmentation for acute ischemic stroke using non-contrast computed tomography. Int. J. Comput. Assist. Radiol. Surg. **17**(4), 661–671 (2022)
5. Mehrtash, A., Wells, W.M., Tempany, C.M., Abolmaesumi, P., Kapur, T.: Confidence calibration and predictive uncertainty estimation for deep medical image segmentation. IEEE Trans. Med. Imaging **39**(12), 3868–3878 (2020)
6. Öman, O., Mäkelä, T., Salli, E., Savolainen, S., Kangasniemi, M.: 3D convolutional neural networks applied to CT angiography in the detection of acute ischemic stroke. European Radiol. Experimental **3**, 1–11 (2019)
7. Ostmeier, S., et al.: Random expert sampling for deep learning segmentation of acute ischemic stroke on non-contrast CT. arXiv:2309.03930 (2023)
8. Tsao, C.W., et al.: Heart disease and stroke statistics-2023 update: a report from the American Heart association. Circulation **147**(8), e93–e621 (2023)
9. Vorberg, L., Taubmann, O., Ditt, H., Maier, A.: Segmentation of acute ischemic stroke in native and enhanced CT using uncertainty-aware labels. In: BVM Workshop. pp. 267–272. Springer (2024). https://doi.org/10.1007/978-3-658-44037-4_72
10. de Vries, L., Emmer, B.J., Majoie, C.B., Marquering, H.A., Gavves, E.: PerfU-net: baseline infarct estimation from CT perfusion source data for acute ischemic stroke. Med. Image Anal. **85**, 102749 (2023)
11. Zhao, Y., Yang, C., Schweidtmann, A., Tao, Q.: Efficient bayesian uncertainty estimation for nnU-Net. In: International Conference on Medical Image Computing and Computer-Assisted Intervention, pp. 535–544. Springer (2022). https://doi.org/10.1007/978-3-031-16452-1_51
12. Zou, K., Chen, Z., Yuan, X., Shen, X., Wang, M., Fu, H.: A review of uncertainty estimation and its application in medical imaging. Meta-Radiol., 100003 (2023)

# Usefulness of Monoenergetic Non-contrast CT and X-Map Images for Deep Learning-Based Stroke Lesion Segmentation

Linda Vorberg[1,2]([✉]) [iD], Hendrik Ditt[2] [iD], Michael Sühling[2] [iD], Andreas Maier[1] [iD], Nicolas Murray[3] [iD], Savvas Nicolaou[3] [iD], and Oliver Taubmann[2] [iD]

[1] Friedrich-Alexander-Universität Erlangen-Nürnberg, Erlangen, Germany
linda.vorberg@fau.de
[2] CT R&D Image Analytics, Siemens Healthineers, Forchheim, Germany
[3] Department of Radiology, Vancouver General Hospital,
University of British Columbia, Vancouver, Canada

**Abstract.** This study investigates the usefulness of monoenergetic non-contrast computed tomography (NCCT) and x-map images in comparison to conventional NCCT for neural network-based stroke lesion segmentation. Utilizing the nnU-Net segmentation framework, models are trained on conventional, Mono+50, Mono+70, and Mono+120 NCCT as well as x-map images. Performance is evaluated on all image types, including those not seen during training, with the network predicting stroke core and hypoperfused volumes. Evaluation metrics include Dice scores and volumetric measurements. Results indicate that training nnU-Net with Mono+120 images on average yields the best performance across all tested image types. While x-map images, previously shown to facilitate lesion detection in human reader studies, do not outperform Mono+120 in same-domain training and testing, they demonstrate robust performance in inference for different energy level and conventional NCCT-trained models. For medium sized infarcts of 10–70 ml, the best Dice score is achieved when training with Mono+120 and testing on x-map images. These findings highlight the potential benefits of advanced spectral CT image derivatives for ischemic stroke segmentation.

**Keywords:** Stroke Segmentation · Spectral CT · Dual Energy CT

## 1 Introduction

Stroke remains a major global health challenge and the second leading cause of death, with ischemic strokes accounting for 62.4% of all stroke cases [10]. To exclude hemorrhage, a non-contrast CT scan (NCCT) is acquired as a first-line imaging tool. It is characterized by its wide-spread availability and rapid acquisition. Subsequent CT Angiography (CTA) and CT Perfusion reveal more

R. Su et al. (Eds.): ISLES 2024/SWITCH 2024, LNCS 15408, pp. 31–39, 2025.
https://doi.org/10.1007/978-3-031-81101-2_4

sophisticated insights into the status of blood supply in the brain. Nevertheless, ischemic changes may already be visible on the NCCT scan, due to increased water uptake in infarcted areas, but may be subtle and hard to detect [6].

Spectral imaging techniques such as dual-energy CT (DECT) and photon-counting CT (PCCT) utilize information from different X-ray energy levels, which allows to generate virtual monoenergetic images with enhanced contrast, reduced noise or mitigated beam hardening artifacts, depending on the choice of energy level [1]. Additionally, there is a rather novel image type, derived from dual energy NCCT – x-map – designed for stroke detection purposes. A suppression of bone and fat combined with a reduction of gray-white matter contrast is achieved using the three material decomposition technique [7]. In this way, edema signals, marking the increased water uptake of the tissue, make ischemic changes easier to detect. In recent work, human reader studies have shown the benefit of x-map images over conventional NCCT in the identification of ischemic lesions in the brain. Noguchi et al. compared lesion detection using x-map against simulated 120 keV NCCT images of 6 patients [7]. The sensitivity using x-map was superior to standard CT and the lesions, characterized by areas of low attenuation in the x-map, correlated well with the findings on DWI MRI scans. To enhance and speed up the diagnostic process of stroke identification and subsequent treatment planning, Deep Learning (DL) models have been employed for stroke classification and segmentation. Wang et al. used a SwinUNETR, combining a self-attention-based encoder with a convolution-based decoder, for the automated delineation of ischemic lesions on NCCT [11]. They achieved a Dice score of 46.7% against expert-annotated DWI ground truth labels. The average difference in lesion volume between prediction and ground truth was 27.1 ml, while the median lesion size in the test cohort was 35.2 ml.

While previous studies have highlighted the potential of automated assessments in improving diagnostic speed and accuracy, the effectiveness of DL models with x-map images remains unexplored. This study aims to assess the advantages of using monoenergetic and x-map images over conventional NCCT images in stroke segmentation. Given the proven advantage of x-map images in human reader studies, we investigate how the nnUNet segmentation framework can leverage these images to enhance stroke segmentation.

## 2   Materials and Methods

### 2.1   Data

The dataset used in this work was acquired at a single site, Vancouver General Hospital, and comprises CT scans of 96 patients. These include NCCT, CTA and CT Perfusion, all acquired with a Somatom Force (Siemens Healthineers, Forchheim, Germany) DECT scanner. For the purposes of network training, only NCCT images were employed. These scans were acquired at tube voltages of 90 and 150 kV and have a size of $512 \times 512$ pixels and an average voxel spacing of $0.45 \times 0.45 \times 0.99 \, mm^3$. CT Perfusion scans (original resolution $0.41 \times 0.41 \times 2.98 \, mm^3$) were utilized to facilitate the annotation process based on perfusion maps that encode Cerebral Blood Volume (CBV), Cerebral Blood Flow (CBF), and Time to Maximum Enhancement (TMAX). Additionally, if a follow-up MRI was available (26 patients), it was also taken into account during the annotation process comparing the localization of the lesion with the perfusion maps. Out of the total cohort, 20 patients exhibited a prior infarct. The mean size of acute infarcts (90 patients) being $13.3 \pm 18.0$ ml. In the remaining 6 patients, only prior infarcts could be identified but all 96 cases available were used in this study.

## 2.2  Labeling Scheme

The annotated labels consider the uncertainty inherent to the task of stroke lesion segmentation. Disparities between expert annotators exist in the context of medical image segmentation [5] and are particularly evident in the delineation of stroke lesions, where perfusion maps generated from CT Perfusion are used clinically to assess the extent of penumbra and infarct core before treatment. These maps allow considerable interpretative variability and common threshold-based techniques for delineating the affected tissue are prone to artifacts and therefore not suitable as a reliable reference standard per se. Therefore, uncertainty-aware labels are used in this study to pragmatically capture uncertainty by defining an inner and outer boundary for stroke core and hypoperfused volume, which is defined as the union of core and surrounding penumbra. The inner contour encodes the minimum assumed extent which should be completely covered by the prediction while the outer boundary represents the maximum presumed extent beyond which the entity would be considered oversegmented. Combining annotations of multiple experts would also allow the construction of the described label scheme, but in this work one annotator used CBV, CBF and TMAX maps to derive the boundaries. Figure 1a shows an example for a label, with a tube-like structure forming an area of "uncertainty," as the inner boundary is always enclosed by the outer boundary of the segmented tissue. As an auxiliary training task, a single label for prior infarcts is provided to the segmentation network to separate them from acute infarctions. The NCCT images used for network training are registered and resampled to the baseline time point of the perfusion, on which the labels were created. Beforehand, the perfusion images are upsampled to a voxel spacing of $0.41 \times 0.41 \times 1.0\,\mathrm{mm}^3$ to preserve information from the higher resolution NCCT data.

## 2.3  Generation of Monoenergetic and X-Map Images

To explore the benefits of spectral CT for stroke segmentation, virtual monoenergetic images at different levels and so called x-map images were used and compared in this study. With a DECT scanner, two images are acquired simultaneously at different energy levels, in this case at 90 and 150 kV, which allows for material decomposition and the creation of virtual monoenergetic images [4]. These monoenergetic images mimic the acquisition of a scan at a certain energy level. Monoenergetic images at levels of 50 keV, 70 keV and 120 keV as well as a mixed image that is equivalent to a conventional CT image were calculated.

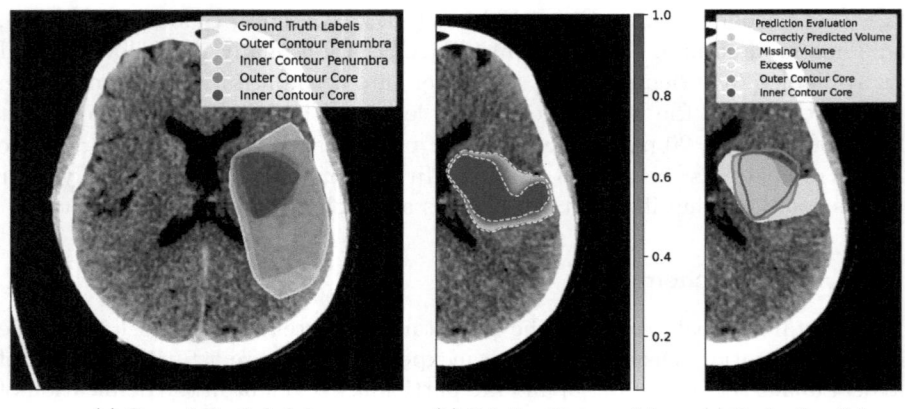

(a) Ground Truth Labels    (b) Relative Distance Map    (c) Evaluation Scheme

**Fig. 1.** Figure 1a: Ground truth of core and penumbra with inner and outer boundary overlay on NCCT. Figure 1b: Result of post-processed prediction of core resulting in relative distance. Figure 1c: Prediction shown in Fig. 1b thresholded at 0.5 and compared to ground truth labels of infarct core (same contours as in Fig. 1a).

Lower keV offers the benefit of enhanced contrast but also comes with increased noise, whereas high keV generates less noisy images [2]. Additionally, x-map images are derived from the dual energy NCCT scan. X-map reduces gray-white matter contrast and removes fat and bone from the image. It is therefore supposed to increase detectability of ischemic lesions [7]. An example of all image types used in the following experiments is shown in the upper row of Fig. 3.

## 2.4   Experiment Setup

We employed the nnU-Net framework as our segmentation network [3]. It is a self-configuring framework that is state-of-the-art for medical image segmentation. For this purpose, the 3D full-resolution variant of nnU-Net was trained over 1000 epochs. As the labels described above follow a hierarchical order (inner boundary is enclosed by the outer boundary and core is surrounded by penumbra), the region-based training feature of nnU-Net was employed. This enables the network to learn regions of merged labels rather than individual labels. Separate instances of nnU-Net models were trained, exclusively using data from a single image type as input for each model. All models were trained using a five-fold cross validation scheme, which is separate from the train/validation split utilized in nnU-Net's internal cross-validation. This approach allows us to acquire averaged test statistics across all cases, providing a comprehensive evaluation of the model's performance. To further investigate the generalizability of monoenergetic and x-map images, cross-inference is performed by inferring all samples of an image type on the models trained on the other domains.

## 2.5   Evaluation

**Post-processing.** Based on the network output a set of possible delineations of both core and hypoperfused volume can be derived. To this end, the Euclidean Distance Transform (EDT) [9] is calculated for every voxel $x$ within the area between inner and outer boundary,

$$d_k(x) = \min_{y \in \Omega_k} \left( \|x - y\|_2 \right), k \in \{O, I\}. \tag{1}$$

Hereby, the distance to the nearest voxel $(y)$ located in the inner $(d_I)$ and outside the outer boundary $(d_O)$ is calculated, with $\Omega_k$ describing the respective set of voxels. The relative distance $d_r \in [0, 1]$,

$$d_r(x) = \frac{d_O(x)}{d_O(x) + d_I(x)}, \tag{2}$$

is depicted in Fig. 1b and can be thresholded to obtain a single contour determining the extent of the lesion.

**Evaluation Metrics.** For each distance, the resulting binary mask is compared to the ground truth labels which delineate inner and outer boundaries of the tissue. We evaluate the missing volume, defined as the area within the inner ground truth contour that was not predicted, and the excess volume, which consists of predicted areas outside the outer contour. The intersection between the predicted mask and the region encompassed by inner and outer label is counted as correctly predicted volume. These three volumetric measurements are depicted in Fig. 1c. Utilizing this pattern, we compute a modified Dice coefficient,

$$D(A, B_I, B_O) = \frac{2 \cdot |A \cap B_O|}{|A| + |B_I| + |A \cap (B_O \setminus B_I)|}. \tag{3}$$

$A$, $B_I$ and $B_O$ denote the prediction and the regions enclosed by the inner and outer boundary, respectively. While slightly overestimating larger predictions within $B_O$, this measure remains closely aligned with the original Dice score.

## 3   Results

The cases are divided into four subgroups according to the ground truth volume of the infarct core: <1 ml, 1–10 ml, 10–70 ml, and >70 ml. Consistent with the protocol described in [8], patients whose infarct volume was under 1 ml were deemed clinically irrelevant and thus omitted from our analysis. Consequently, this resulted in a cohort of 73 patients distributed across the remaining three subgroups, with 46 patients in the 1–10 ml subgroup, 25 in the 10–70 ml subgroup, and 2 in the subgroup exceeding 70 ml. The relative distance map derived from the predicted labels is thresholded at distinct levels ranging from 0.0 to 1.0 in steps of 0.1, while in the following, only the result for the threshold yielding

**Table 1.** Average (± std) of missing and excess volume for experiments using the same image type for model **training**. Results are given per volume group.

| Training Dataset | Missing Volume (ml) | | | Excess Volume (ml) | | |
|---|---|---|---|---|---|---|
| | 1–10 ml | 10–70 ml | >70 ml | 1–10 ml | 10–70 ml | >70 ml |
| Mixed | 2.8 ± 0.1 | 15.4 ± 0.8 | 73.0 ± 2.2 | 2.9 ± 0.9 | 2.7 ± 1.2 | 0.7 ± 0.5 |
| Mono+50 | 2.9 ± 0.1 | 16.3 ± 0.6 | 76.5 ± 1.6 | 1.8 ± 0.5 | 1.5 ± 1.0 | 0.4 ± 0.5 |
| Mono+70 | 2.8 ± 0.1 | 15.6 ± 0.6 | 74.7 ± 1.9 | 2.4 ± 1.8 | 2.4 ± 1.9 | 0.3 ± 0.2 |
| Mono+120 | 2.8 ± 0.1 | 15.1 ± 0.7 | 73.0 ± 2.1 | 3.1 ± 0.7 | 3.0 ± 0.8 | 0.7 ± 0.5 |
| x-map | 2.9 ± 0.1 | 16.1 ± 0.9 | 73.7 ± 4.3 | 1.3 ± 1.0 | 1.0 ± 1.1 | 0.3 ± 0.3 |

**Table 2.** Average (± std) of missing and excess volume for experiments using the same image type for **inference**. Results are given per volume group.

| Inference Dataset | Missing Volume (ml) | | | Excess Volume (ml) | | |
|---|---|---|---|---|---|---|
| | 1–10 ml | 10–70 ml | >70 ml | 1–10 ml | 10–70 ml | >70 ml |
| Mixed | 2.8 ± 0.1 | 15.6 ± 0.6 | 74.1 ± 1.7 | 2.3 ± 0.8 | 1.8 ± 0.8 | 0.8 ± 0.5 |
| Mono+50 | 2.9 ± 0.1 | 16.2 ± 0.6 | 75.8 ± 1.6 | 1.7 ± 0.9 | 2.3 ± 1.5 | 0.1 ± 0.1 |
| Mono+70 | 2.9 ± 0.1 | 15.8 ± 0.9 | 75.0 ± 2.9 | 2.0 ± 1.3 | 2.0 ± 1.6 | 0.5 ± 0.5 |
| Mono+120 | 2.8 ± 0.1 | 15.9 ± 0.9 | 73.0 ± 4.0 | 1.7 ± 0.7 | 1.1 ± 0.7 | 0.4 ± 0.4 |
| x-map | 2.8 ± 0.1 | 15.0 ± 0.7 | 73.0 ± 2.7 | 3.7 ± 1.3 | 3.4 ± 1.3 | 0.6 ± 0.3 |

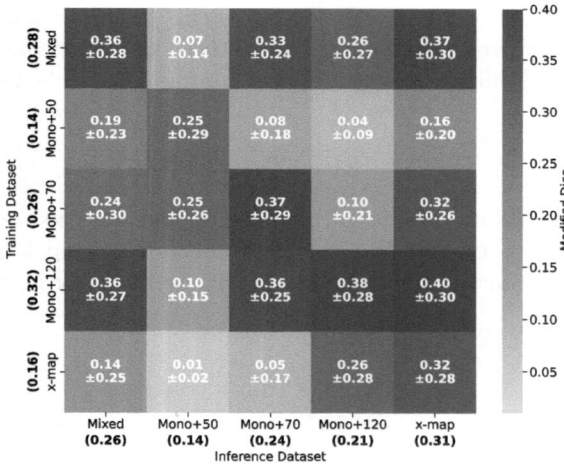

**Fig. 2.** Average (± std) modified Dice for volume group 10–70 ml. The numbers in parens denote the average modified Dice per row or column.

the best modified Dice score in each experiment is presented. Figure 2 shows the average modified Dice across all experiments performed for the cases of the

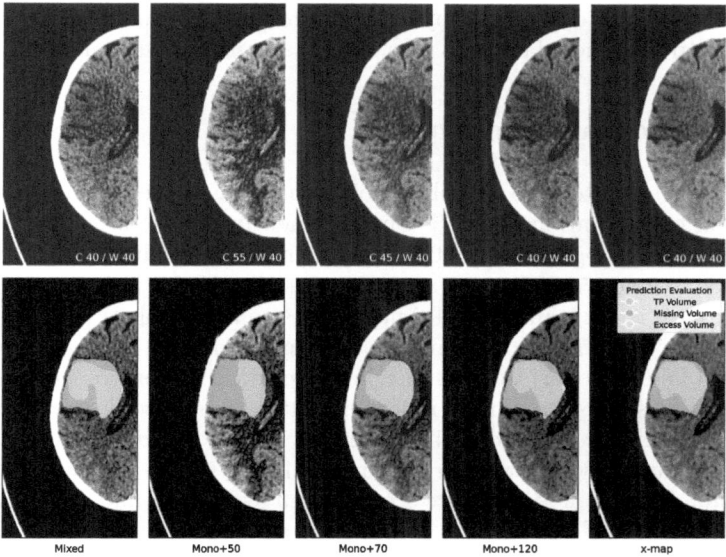

**Fig. 3.** Qualitative comparisons. TP denotes correctly predicted volume.

10–70 ml subgroup as this is considered the most relevant group. The diagonal represents training and testing on images from the same image type, while all other fields show the results for cross-inference. The best modified Dice value for in-domain experiments for this volume group is 0.38 for Mono+120 images, but this performance can be improved to 0.40 when using x-map images for inference on the same model. It can be seen that a model trained on Mono+120 images exhibits the best results, reflected by the mean value of the row of the heatmap. Compared to the other models, x-map training does not show superior performance when used for training, but has the best average values across all the models for inference. This trend can also be observed considering the assessment of missing and excess predicted volume. The averaged volumetric measurements are shown in Table 1 and Table 2 for all volume groups. Table 1 also demonstrates the superiority of training with Mono+120 images regarding missing volume. Across all volume groups, the Mono+120 model yields values lower or on par with the other models. Excess volume for the Mono+120 model is slightly higher than for the remaining models but still relatively small with e.g., 15.1 ml of missing volume vs. 3.0 ml of excess volume for infarcts in the 10–70 ml subgroup. Similar results are observed for the averaged volumetric measures across the inference datasets in Table 2. Supporting the tendency seen in the Dice score, inference on x-map images for different models yields the lowest missing volumes across the different volume groups. As before, excess volume is slightly higher for x-map but still low compared to the values for missing volume.

Figure 3 presents qualitative results from models trained and tested on the same image type. The upper row displays the original images. In the lower row, the predicted stroke core is overlayed, highlighting both the missing and excess predicted regions. The infarct was identified in all images but to different extents.

## 4   Discussion and Conclusion

This work investigates the usefulness of monoenergetic and x-map images in comparison to conventional NCCT when segmenting stroke lesions using a neural network. As a segmentation framework, nnU-Net is employed and trained with mixed, Mono+50, Mono+70 and Mono+120 NCCT images as well as x-map. Inference is performed on all image types to also explore the performance on a "domain" that has not been seen during training. The network predicts stroke core and hypoperfused volume, incorporating regions of uncertainty by leveraging labels consisting of an inner and outer boundary. For evaluation, the area between the two predicted boundaries is transformed into a relative distance map that allows for the derivation of different lesion extents by applying a threshold. A mean modified Dice score as well as missing and excess predicted volumes are reported by comparison with the ground truth label.

Training with Mono+120 images yields the best average performance. X-map, which was shown to make lesions easier to detect in reader studies, is not superior to Mono+120 when training/testing is performed on the same image type. However, x-map demonstrates the best performance across all trained models when the inference image type is fixed. Conversely, training on x-map typically yields inferior performance when inference is done with other image types. We assume that this is due to the fact x-map is designed to suppress physiological characteristics that may be misidentified as infarction: If the model has not seen these during training, it will not be able to assess them correctly during inference. However, when the model is exposed to them during training, they serve as difficulty augmentation and do not hurt performance as long as image appearance is comparable, i.e. the "domain" shift between training and inference is negligible. This is the case with high energy images as these similarly reduce the gray/white matter contrast. In fact, training with Mono+120 images and testing x-map yields the best Dice score of 0.4 for the 10–70 ml volume group , which is roughly comparable to the results achieved by Wang et al. [11]. The modified Dice incorporates tolerance from uncertainty-aware labeling, which typically yields somewhat higher scores, yet mean lesion volume in [11] is larger (35.2 ml) than the average volume in our 10–70 ml subgroup (23.4 ml), which is also conducive to a better performance. In general, infarcts were rather underestimated, proven by the higher values of missing volume compared to excess volume. Mono+50 images showed the worst performance, for both training and inference. These images exhibit a very high contrast between gray and white matter, which is also seen in the qualitative results (Fig. 3). While visible, the infarct is harder to distinguish from surrounding tissue and accordingly only a smaller part is detected by the model.

Overall, benefits of spectral image types are moderate compared to conventional CT. Based on our results, it appears there is no significant downside to training a model on conventional images, which are more readily available, and using this at inference time with either conventional images—when spectral information is not available or the typical image appearance is preferred—or the task-specific x-map visualization, both at similar levels of model performance only slightly below the optimum that relies on Mono+120 images for training.

In conclusion, our observations provide insights into the potential of spectral CT for DL-based segmentation of ischemic stroke. However, given the limitations of a single-site dataset, further research is needed to substantiate these findings.

# References

1. D'Angelo, T., et al.: Dual energy computed tomography virtual monoenergetic imaging: technique and clinical applications. Br. J. Radiol. **92**(1098), 20180546 (2019)
2. Grant, K.L., Flohr, T.G., Krauss, B., Sedlmair, M., Thomas, C., Schmidt, B.: Assessment of an advanced image-based technique to calculate virtual monoenergetic computed tomographic images from a dual-energy examination to improve contrast-to-noise ratio in examinations using iodinated contrast media. Invest. Radiol. **49**(9), 586–592 (2014)
3. Isensee, F., Jaeger, P.F., Kohl, S.A., Petersen, J., Maier-Hein, K.H.: nnU-Net: a self-configuring method for deep learning-based biomedical image segmentation. Nat. Methods **18**(2), 203–211 (2021)
4. Johnson, T.R.: Dual-energy CT: general principles. Am. J. Roentgenol. **199**(5_supplement), S3–S8 (2012)
5. Joskowicz, L., Cohen, D., Caplan, N., Sosna, J.: Inter-observer variability of manual contour delineation of structures in CT. Eur. Radiol. **29**, 1391–1399 (2019)
6. Lin, S.Y., Chiang, P.L., Chen, P.W., Cheng, L.H., Chen, M.H., Chang, P.C., Lin, W.C., Chen, Y.S.: Toward automated segmentation for acute ischemic stroke using non-contrast computed tomography. Int. J. Comput. Assist. Radiol. Surg. **17**(4), 661–671 (2022)
7. Noguchi, K., Itoh, T., Naruto, N., Takashima, S., Tanaka, K., Kuroda, S.: A novel imaging technique (X-map) to identify acute ischemic lesions using noncontrast dual-energy computed tomography. J. Stroke Cerebrovasc. Dis. **26**(1), 34–41 (2017)
8. Ostmeier, S., et al.: Random expert sampling for deep learning segmentation of acute ischemic stroke on non-contrast CT. arXiv:2309.03930 (2023)
9. Strutz, T.: The distance transform and its computation. arXiv preprint arXiv:2106.03503 (2021)
10. Tsao, C.W., et al.: Heart disease and stroke statistics-2023 update: a report from the American Heart Association. Circulation **147**(8), e93–e621 (2023)
11. Wang, W.C., et al.: Automated delineation of acute ischemic stroke lesions on non-contrast CT using 3D deep learning: a promising step towards efficient diagnosis and treatment. Biomed. Signal Process. Control **93**, 106139 (2024)

# Improved Stroke Lesion Segmentation via Cross-Model Knowledge Distillation

Zixin Liu, Haowen Pang, Xinru Zhang, and Chuyang Ye$^{(\boxtimes)}$

School of Integrated Circuits and Electronics, Beijing Institute of Technology,
Beijing, China
`chuyang.ye@bit.edu.cn`

**Abstract.** Stroke lesion segmentation is a crucial step in stroke disease analysis as it provides essential anatomical information for the diagnosis and prognosis. Deep learning approaches, including the *convolutional neural network* (CNN) and Transformer, have improved the accuracy of automated stroke lesion segmentation. Since CNN-based models generally learn to extract local features with convolutional filters, whereas Transformer-based models excel in modeling long-range dependencies with self-attention mechanisms, combining the strengths of the two types of models may bring additional benefits. Existing studies have proposed various hybrid network structures combining convolution and self-attention; however, empirical evidence shows that these hybrid structures do not necessarily outperform purely CNN-based or Transformer-based methods. Thus, this work further explores the integration of the strengths of CNNs and Transformers. Instead of constructing a hybrid network architecture, we propose a cross-model interaction method based on knowledge distillation, which can effectively allow CNN-based and Transformer-based models to learn the strength of each other. The guidance is achieved with an adaptive recall-enhancing loss for knowledge distillation, which suppresses negative knowledge transfer and encourages the model to reduce false negative predictions that are common in stroke lesion segmentation. We validated the proposed method on two public stroke lesion segmentation datasets, where it improves the segmentation performance compared with the best competing segmentation model by 2.0% and 1.4% for the ISLES and ATLAS dataset, respectively.

**Keywords:** Stroke lesion segmentation · cross-model interaction · knowledge distillation

## 1 Introduction

Automated stroke lesion segmentation plays an important role in stroke disease analysis [1]. It can provide quantitative measures of stroke lesions, which are crucial information for diagnosis and prognosis [2,25]. However, due to the diverse appearances, fuzzy boundaries, and diffuse locations of stroke lesions, accurate stroke lesion segmentation can be a challenging task. Traditional stroke lesion

R. Su et al. (Eds.): ISLES 2024/SWITCH 2024, LNCS 15408, pp. 40–50, 2025.
https://doi.org/10.1007/978-3-031-81101-2_5

segmentation methods rely on hand-crafted features and machine learning models [5,20], but the feature design may not be optimal for segmentation, and the segmentation performance is usually unsatisfactory. More recent works on stroke lesion segmentation are inspired by the success of *deep learning* (DL) in image processing, where various DL segmentation models are developed [7,17].

Two widely used DL segmentation models include *convolutional neural networks* (CNNs) and Transformers, both of which have been applied to stroke lesion segmentation [6,18]. U-Net [18] is a well-known CNN-based segmentation model that consists of an encoder and a decoder, with skip connections to capture information at different scales. UNet++ improves the segmentation by introducing multi-scale cascading, enhanced skip connections, and dense connections [24]; nnU-Net utilizes the U-Net architecture and achieves optimal performance various stroke lesion segmentation tasks through meticulously designed preprocessing and postprocessing steps [14]. By contrast, Transformer-based models that exploit the self-attention mechanism for modeling long-range dependencies have also achieved promising segmentation performance [8,22]. For example, Swin-Unet is a U-shaped Transformer architecture that takes long-range dependencies into consideration [3]; nnFormer introduces a network architecture that is mainly composed of the Transformer structure, where a Transformer-based stem is used together with convolutional embedding and upsampling/downsampling [23].

Both CNN and Transformer architectures have their own strengths. The use of convolution in CNNs allows the model to emphasize local feature patterns, whereas the use of self-attention in Transformers allows the model to better capture global information. Therefore, it is desirable to combine their merits, and existing research has proposed hybrid frameworks combining CNNs and Transformers. For example, TransUNet is proposed as a CNN-Transformer hybrid network for medical image segmentation, which uses cascaded convolutional and Transformer layers as the encoder and pure convolutional layers as the decoder [6]; UNETR introduces a hybrid architecture with a Transformer-based encoder and a CNN-based decoder, and skip connections are incorporated to fuse the Transformer and CNN outputs at each resolution level [11]; in addition, Swin UNETR is proposed based on the design of UNETR and Swin Transformer [10]. However, since it is challenging to determine the optimal architecture design [15], empirical evidence shows that the hybrid models do not necessarily outperform well-engineered CNN-based or Transformer-based models [14].

In this work, we further explore the problem of integrating CNN-based and Transformer-based models for improving stroke lesion segmentation. Instead of seeking to construct a hybrid architecture, we propose to jointly leverage their strengths with the interaction between these models. The cross-model interaction is achieved with a knowledge distillation framework designed for stroke lesion segmentation. We assume that we have a CNN-based model and a Transformer-based model—one model is considered the teacher model and the other is the student model. The student model learns from both the manual annotation and the prediction of the teacher model. Since previous works have demonstrated that the knowledge in a model can be encoded in its predictions [13], this allows a CNN-based model to acquire the knowledge learned by a Transformer-based model and vice versa. To avoid negative knowledge transfer caused by incorrect predictions of the teacher model, an adaptive knowledge distillation loss is proposed, which suppresses the learning of misleading information. Furthermore, based on the observation that stroke lesion segmentation models tend to miss small lesions [21], the knowledge distillation loss is designed with a focus on recall to reduce false negatives. Moreover, as the knowledge distillation process naturally produces multiple segmentation models, these models can be further ensembled for better segmentation quality. To validate the proposed method, experiments were performed on two public datasets for stroke lesion segmentation. The results show that our method outperforms state-of-the-art CNN-based, Transformer-based, and hybrid segmentation models.

## 2    Methods

### 2.1    Problem Formulation and Method Overview

Suppose we are given a set of training images with stroke lesion annotations. Conventionally, a stroke lesion segmentation model, for example a CNN-based or Transformer-based model, is trained directly based on the annotated data regardless of other models. In this work, we seek to train the CNN-based or Transformer-based model with the guidance of the other model, so that the strengths of CNNs and Transformers can be integrated. More specifically, we assume that one model, the teacher model $\mathcal{M}_t$, has first been trained with the annotated data, and the other model, the student model $\mathcal{M}_s$, is to be trained with both the annotated data and the teacher model guidance. Note that although it may be possible to jointly train the two models with interaction between them, this induces substantially increased computational overhead, which can be impractical due to the GPU memory constraint. The teacher model can be either the CNN-based or Transformer-based model, and the student model is the other type. The key component of the framework is the interaction between the teacher and student models, and its detailed design is given below.

### 2.2    Cross-Model Knowledge Distillation

Since the teacher and student models are based on different types of architectures, i.e., CNN and Transformer, they acquire different knowledge for the same segmentation task. If the knowledge of the teacher model can be transferred to the student model, then the student model combines the strengths of both CNNs and Transformers. Since one common strategy for such knowledge transfer is knowledge distillation [13], we develop our teacher-student interaction framework based on cross-model knowledge distillation.

As it has been previously shown that the knowledge of a model can be encoded in its output [13], our knowledge distillation exploits the prediction $y_t$ of the teacher model $\mathcal{M}_t$. Specifically, the training of the student model $\mathcal{M}_s$ is achieved by minimizing a loss function $\mathcal{L}$ that combines the supervised segmentation loss $\mathcal{L}_{\text{seg}}$ and the knowledge distillation loss $\mathcal{L}_{\text{kd}}$:

$$\mathcal{L}(y, y_{\text{t}}, y_{\text{s}}) = (1 - \alpha)\mathcal{L}_{\text{seg}}(y, y_{\text{s}}) + \alpha\mathcal{L}_{\text{kd}}(y_{\text{t}}, y_{\text{s}}). \tag{1}$$

Here, $y$ is the manual annotation (gold standard), $y_{\text{s}}$ is the prediction of $\mathcal{M}_{\text{s}}$, and $\alpha$ is the weight for loss combination. $\mathcal{L}_{\text{seg}}(y, y_{\text{s}})$ measures the difference between the annotation and the student prediction, whereas $\mathcal{L}_{\text{kd}}(y_{\text{t}}, y_{\text{s}})$ measures the discrepancy between the teacher and student prediction.

$\mathcal{L}_{\text{seg}}(y, y_{\text{s}})$ can be computed with the standard *cross-entropy* (CE) and Dice loss [9]. However, direct computation of $\mathcal{L}_{\text{kd}}(y_{\text{t}}, y_{\text{s}})$ with the CE and Dice loss can be suboptimal for two reasons. First, the teacher model can generate erroneous segmentation results, the learning of which could be harmful to the student model. Second, due to the predominance of the background class, DL models tend to produce false negative stroke lesion segmentation results even with the Dice loss that is less sensitive to the imbalance. As CNN-based and Transformer-based models give different segmentation results, we expect the knowledge distillation to focus on the difference between the lesions correctly detected by the two types of models to reduce the false negatives. However, the CE and Dice loss does not specifically address the problem for stroke lesion segmentation.

To address these issues, we propose an adaptive determination of $\alpha$ and a recall-enhancing knowledge distillation loss for the cross-model interaction. First, instead of setting a constant $\alpha$ value for the contribution of knowledge distillation, we choose to dynamically determine $\alpha$ based on the teacher and student model predictions. We assume that learning from the teacher model is effective when it is more accurate than the student model. The accuracy can be simply measured by the Dice coefficients $D_{\text{t}}$ and $D_{\text{s}}$ of $y_{\text{t}}$ and $y_{\text{s}}$ with respect to $y$, respectively. Then, when the teacher model is not more accurate than the student model, its prediction is ignored by setting $\alpha = 0$, where we have

$$\alpha = \begin{cases} 0 & \text{if } D_{\text{t}} \leq D_{\text{s}} \\ 0.5 & \text{otherwise} \end{cases}. \tag{2}$$

Here, when the teacher model is more accurate than the student model, the contributions of $\mathcal{L}_{\text{seg}}(y, y_{\text{s}})$ and $\mathcal{L}_{\text{kd}}(y_{\text{t}}, y_{\text{s}})$ are the same, which avoids injecting a bias into the model.

Second, $\mathcal{L}_{\text{kd}}(y_{\text{t}}, y_{\text{s}})$ is designed to reduce false negative predictions. We assume that by learning from the lesion voxels that are correctly identified by the teacher model but missed by the student model, the student model is encouraged to leverage knowledge that it may neglect otherwise to reduce false negatives. For example, suppose $\mathcal{M}_{\text{t}}$ is Transformer-based and $\mathcal{M}_{\text{s}}$ is CNN-based. Without the guidance of $\mathcal{M}_{\text{t}}$, $\mathcal{M}_{\text{s}}$ tends to leverage local features instead of global information, which leads to the detection of certain lesion voxels but not others. The detection of lesion voxels that are correctly detected by $\mathcal{M}_{\text{t}}$ but missed by $\mathcal{M}_{\text{s}}$ requires more global information. By forcing $\mathcal{M}_{\text{s}}$ to find these lesion voxels, the CNN is encouraged to learn global knowledge or extract features that are equivalent to the global information. This knowledge distillation allows the student model to exploit the strengths of both CNN-based and Transformer-based models and enhances the recall of the segmentation result. Mathematically, the recall-enhancing knowledge distillation loss is defined as a masked CE loss:

$$\mathcal{L}_{\mathrm{kd}}(y, y_{\mathrm{t}}, y_{\mathrm{s}}) = \sum_i m^i y_{\mathrm{t}}^i \log y_{\mathrm{s}}^i, \qquad (3)$$

where $y^i$, $y_{\mathrm{t}}^i$, and $y_{\mathrm{s}}^i$ represent the annotation, teacher prediction, and student prediction at the $i$-th voxel, respectively, and $m^i$ is a binary indicator that is one when both the annotation and teacher prediction suggest that the $i$-th voxel belongs to the lesion and zero otherwise.

### 2.3   Model Ensembling

The cross-model interaction naturally provides multiple segmentation models. Both the CNN-based and Transformer-based models can be used as the student model or the teacher model, which leads to a CNN-based teacher model, a Transformer-based teacher model, a CNN-based student model, and a Transformer-based student model. These models produce segmentation results with different focuses on the image information. Thus, we expect that their predictions are complementary and integrate the segmentation results of all four trained models. A simple majority voting strategy is used to ensemble the segmentation results, and a voxel is considered background with tied votes.

### 2.4   Implementation Details

We choose nnU-Net [14] as the CNN-based model and nnFormer [23] the Transformer-based model, as these two models are representative and have achieved superior segmentation performance compared with alternative models. nnU-Net and nnFormer can automatically determine data configurations, such as intensity normalization, the choice between 2D and 3D processing, patch size, batch size, etc. In this work, the same 3D processing was selected by both nnU-Net and nnFormer. The default hyperparameters of nnU-Net and nnFormer were used, except that the number of training epochs was set to a smaller value 200, as we observed that it was sufficient for convergent training.

## 3   Experiments

### 3.1   Data Description

To evaluate the proposed method, experiments were performed on two publicly available datasets for stroke lesion segmentation. The first dataset is the ISLES dataset [12] for acute ischemic stroke lesion segmentation. ISLES comprises 250 annotated *diffusion weighted images* (DWIs) with an isotropic image resolution of 2 mm. The second dataset is the ATLAS dataset [16] for chronic stroke lesion segmentation. ATLAS comprises 655 annotated T1-weighted images, which have the same voxel size of 1 mm isotropic.

For the ISLES/ATLAS dataset, 100/100 images were used as the training set, 25/25 images were used as the validation set for model selection, and 125/530 images were used as the test set, respectively.

## 3.2   Competing Methods

To demonstrate the benefit of the proposed method, we compared our method with the standard nnU-Net and nnFormer (trained without cross-model interaction with the same hyperparameter settings of the proposed method and except for the number of training epochs, all default hyperparameters of nnU-Net or nnFormer are used.). As ensembling can boost the performance of stroke lesion segmentation [19], we also compared our method with the fused results of nnU-Net and nnFormer. In addition, we considered several other representative CNN-based, Transformer-based, and hybrid models for comparison. The additional CNN-based models include the U-Net [18] and UNet++ [24] models implemented in the MONAI framework (Version 2.0) [4], the additional Transformer-based model is Swin-Unet [3] with its open-source implementation, and the additional hybrid models are UNETR [11] and Swin UNETR [10] that are also implemented in MONAI. These models have been widely used in medical image segmentation with excellent performance.

## 3.3   Evaluation Results

We first qualitatively evaluated the proposed method. The segmentation result is overlaid on the input image and shown in a cross-sectional view in Fig. 1. Here, we compared the results of the student models with those of the teacher models. For convenience, the student model is denoted by "nnFormer→nnU-Net" when nnFormer is the teacher model and nnU-Net is the student model, and by "nnU-Net→nnFormer" when nnU-Net is the teacher model and nnFormer is the student model. Compared with the standard nnU-Net and nnFormer, the nnFormer→nnU-Net and nnU-Net→nnFormer models produce segmentation results that better resemble the annotation with reduced false negatives.

Next, we present the quantitative evaluation of our method. The Dice coefficient was computed for the segmentation result on each test scan, and the mean and *standard deviation* (std) of the Dice coefficient are summarized for each method and each dataset in Table 1. For both datasets, either nnU-Net or nnFormer has the best performance among the standard CNN-based, Transformer-based, and hybrid models, which justifies their use in our method. Their ensembled result is better than the individual result for ATLAS but not for ISLES.

Compared with nnU-Net and nnFormer, nnFormer→nnU-Net and nnU-Net→nnFormer respectively have higher Dice coefficients. The segmentation performance is improved by 1.9%/0.9% and 1.4%/0.6% for the ISLES and ATLAS

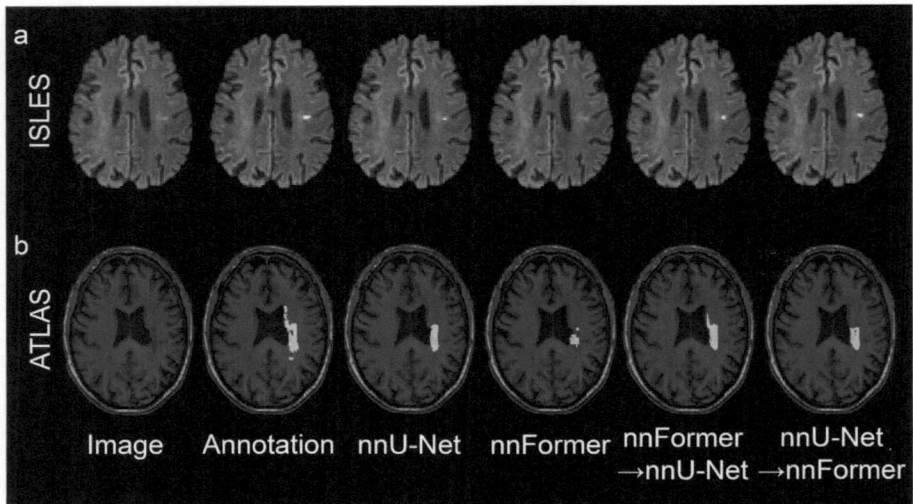

**Fig. 1.** Cross-sectional views of representative segmentation results (red) for (a) ISLES and (b) ATLAS. "nnFormer→nnU-Net"/"nnU-Net→nnFormer" refers to the case where nnFormer/nnU-Net is the teacher model and nnU-Net/nnFormer is the student model, respectively. (Color figure online)

dataset, respectively, which indicates the effectiveness of the proposed cross-model interaction. Note that the cross-model distillation is also better than self-distillation (nnU-Net→nnU-Net and nnFormer→nnFormer). The ensembling of the four teacher and student models consistently achieves the best segmentation accuracy in all cases, and its improvement over the competing methods is statistically significant with the Wilcoxon signed-rank test. compared with nnU-Net/nnFormer, the segmentation performance is improved by 2.0%/8.8% and 5.5%/2.4% for the ISLES and ATLAS dataset, respectively; Compared with the ensembled results of nnU-Net and nnFormer, the segmentation performance is improved by 2.5% and 1.4% for the ISLES and ATLAS dataset, respectively.

Moreover, we calculated the recall values on the ISLES and ATLAS datasets. For the ISLES dataset, the recall values of nnU-Net and nnFormer are 74.05% and 69.78%, respectively, whereas the recall values of nnFormer→nnU-Net and nnU-Net→nnFormer are 76.45% and 69.90%, respectively. For the ATLAS dataset, the recall values of nnU-Net and nnFormer are 52.17% and 54.30%, respectively, whereas the recall values of nnFormer→nnU-Net and nnU-Net→nnFormer are 53.80% and 55.68%, respectively. These results show that the recall is indeed improved with the recall-enhancing knowledge distillation loss.

To further demonstrate the benefit of the proposed design of knowledge distillation, including the adaptive determination of the loss weight and the recall-enhancing loss, we performed additional experiments on the ISLES dataset,

**Table 1.** The Dice coefficients (%) in the format of mean ± std on the test set for each dataset and each method. The best results are highlighted in bold. The proposed method that ensembles the four teacher and student models and each competing method were compared with the Wilcoxon signed-rank test. ($^*$ : $p < 0.05$, $^{**}$ : $p < 0.01$, $^{***}$ : $p < 0.001$)

| Architecture | Method | ISLES | ATLAS |
|---|---|---|---|
| CNN | U-Net | $74.06 \pm 23.09^{***}$ | $51.41 \pm 31.14^{***}$ |
| | UNet++ | $59.58 \pm 30.02^{***}$ | $49.62 \pm 30.67^{***}$ |
| | nnU-Net | $76.35 \pm 22.28^{***}$ | $53.32 \pm 31.57^{***}$ |
| Transformer | Swin-Unet | $37.76 \pm 31.96^{***}$ | $35.74 \pm 28.69^{***}$ |
| | nnFormer | $71.62 \pm 24.05^{***}$ | $54.92 \pm 30.35^{*}$ |
| Hybrid | UNETR | $70.13 \pm 24.83^{***}$ | $35.42 \pm 28.96^{***}$ |
| | Swin UNETR | $74.91 \pm 22.30^{***}$ | $47.83 \pm 31.30^{***}$ |
| Ensemble | nnU-Net+nnFormer | $76.02 \pm 21.11^{***}$ | $55.45 \pm 30.78^{***}$ |
| Our method | nnU-Net→nnU-Net | $77.31 \pm 21.28$ | $53.67 \pm 31.02$ |
| | nnFormer→nnU-Net | $77.79 \pm 20.67$ | $54.06 \pm 30.78$ |
| | nnFormer→nnFormer | $70.81 \pm 23.97$ | $54.83 \pm 30.12$ |
| | nnU-Net→nnFormer | $72.25 \pm 23.82$ | $55.27 \pm 29.55$ |
| | Ensemble of four models | $\mathbf{77.91 \pm 20.77}$ | $\mathbf{56.23 \pm 30.36}$ |

where different knowledge distillation strategies were used. First, the naive use of the CE and Dice loss for knowledge distillation was considered. Second, we replaced the adaptive weight with the constant weight of 0.5 and kept the recall-enhancing loss. Third, the recall-enhancing loss was replaced by the CE and Dice loss and the adaptive weight was retained. The results are shown in Table 2, where the results achieved without any knowledge distillation and with the proposed cross-model interaction are shown again for reference. The individual use of the adaptive weight and the recall-enhancing loss both leads to better segmentation accuracy compared with no knowledge distillation and the CE and Dice loss for knowledge distillation. The combination of the two contributions in the proposed method further improves the performance. These results show that the adaptive determination of the loss weight and the recall-enhancing loss are both beneficial to the segmentation.

**Table 2.** The mean Dice coefficient achieved with different knowledge distillation strategies on the ISLES dataset. The best results are highlighted in bold.

| Knowledge Distillation | nnFormer→nnU-Net | nnU-Net→nnFormer |
|---|---|---|
| N/A | 76.35 | 71.62 |
| CE and Dice loss | 77.01 | 69.72 |
| Recall-enhancing loss | 77.24 | 71.88 |
| Adaptive weight | 77.04 | 71.86 |
| Proposed | **77.79** | **72.25** |

## 4 Conclusion

We have proposed a cross-model interaction method that integrates the strengths of CNN-based and Transformer-based models for improved stroke lesion segmentation. The interaction is achieved with adaptive recall-enhancing knowledge distillation, which suppresses negative knowledge transfer and reduces false negative predictions. It also naturally produces multiple segmentation models, which can be ensembled for further improvement. Experimental results on two stroke lesion segmentation tasks show that our method effectively improves the segmentation accuracy compared with state-of-the-art segmentation models.

## References

1. Barber, P.A., Demchuk, A.M., Zhang, J., Buchan, A.M.: Validity and reliability of a quantitative computed tomography score in predicting outcome of hyperacute stroke before thrombolytic therapy. The Lancet **355**(9216), 1670–1674 (2000)
2. Bonkhoff, A.K., et al.: Outcome after acute ischemic stroke is linked to sex-specific lesion patterns. Nat. Commun. **12**(1), 3289 (2021)
3. Cao, H., Wang, Y., Chen, J., Jiang, D., Zhang, X., Tian, Q., Wang, M.: Swin-Unet: Unet-like pure transformer for medical image segmentation. In: European Conference on Computer Vision, pp. 205–218. Springer (2022). https://doi.org/10.1007/978-3-031-25066-8_9https://github.com/HuCaoFighting/Swin-Unet
4. Cardoso, M.J., et al.: MONAI: an open-source framework for deep learning in healthcare. arXiv preprint arXiv:2211.02701 (2022), https://github.com/Project-MONAI/MONAI
5. Cerri, S., et al.: A contrast-adaptive method for simultaneous whole-brain and lesion segmentation in multiple sclerosis. Neuroimage **225**, 117471 (2021)
6. Chen, J., et al.: TransUnet: transformers make strong encoders for medical image segmentation. arXiv preprint arXiv:2102.04306 (2021)
7. Chen, L.C., Yang, Y., Wang, J., Xu, W., Yuille, A.L.: Attention to scale: scale-aware semantic image segmentation. In: Proceedings of the IEEE Conference on Computer Vision and Pattern Recognition, pp. 3640–3649 (2016)
8. Dosovitskiy, A., et al.: An image is worth 16x16 words: Transformers for image recognition at scale. arXiv preprint arXiv:2010.11929 (2020)

9. Galdran, A., Carneiro, G., Ballester, M.A.G.: On the optimal combination of cross-entropy and soft Dice losses for lesion segmentation with out-of-distribution robustness. In: Diabetic Foot Ulcers Grand Challenge, pp. 40–51. Springer (2022). https://doi.org/10.1007/978-3-031-26354-5_4

10. Hatamizadeh, A., Nath, V., Tang, Y., Yang, D., Roth, H.R., Xu, D.: Swin UNETR: swin transformers for semantic segmentation of brain tumors in MRI images. In: MICCAI Brainlesion Workshop. pp. 272–284. Springer (2021). https://doi.org/10.1007/978-3-031-08999-2_22

11. Hatamizadeh, A., et al.: UNETR: transformers for 3D medical image segmentation. In: Proceedings of the IEEE/CVF Winter Conference on Applications of Computer Vision, pp. 574–584 (2022)

12. Hernandez Petzsche, M.R., et al.: ISLES 2022: a multi-center magnetic resonance imaging stroke lesion segmentation dataset. Sci. Data 9(1), 762 (2022)

13. Hinton, G., Vinyals, O., Dean, J.: Distilling the knowledge in a neural network. arXiv preprint arXiv:1503.02531 (2015)

14. Isensee, F., Jaeger, P.F., Kohl, S.A., Petersen, J., Maier-Hein, K.H.: nnU-Net: a self-configuring method for deep learning-based biomedical image segmentation. Nat. Methods 18(2), 203–211 (2021). https://github.com/MIC-DKFZ/nnUNet

15. Li, C., et al.: BossNAS: exploring hybrid CNN-Transformers with block-wisely self-supervised neural architecture search. In: Proceedings of the IEEE/CVF International Conference on Computer Vision, pp. 12281–12291 (2021)

16. Liew, S.L., et al.: A large, curated, open-source stroke neuroimaging dataset to improve lesion segmentation algorithms. Scientific Data 9(1), 320 (2022)

17. Long, J., Shelhamer, E., Darrell, T.: Fully convolutional networks for semantic segmentation. In: Proceedings of the IEEE Conference on Computer Vision and Pattern Recognition, pp. 3431–3440 (2015)

18. Ronneberger, O., Fischer, P., Brox, T.: U-Net: convolutional networks for biomedical image segmentation. In: Navab, N., Hornegger, J., Wells, W.M., Frangi, A.F. (eds.) MICCAI 2015. LNCS, vol. 9351, pp. 234–241. Springer, Cham (2015). https://doi.org/10.1007/978-3-319-24574-4_28

19. de la Rosa, E., et al.: A robust ensemble algorithm for ischemic stroke lesion segmentation: Generalizability and clinical utility beyond the isles challenge. arXiv preprint arXiv:2403.19425 (2024)

20. Shiee, N., Bazin, P.L., Ozturk, A., Reich, D.S., Calabresi, P.A., Pham, D.L.: A topology-preserving approach to the segmentation of brain images with multiple sclerosis lesions. Neuroimage 49(2), 1524–1535 (2010)

21. Shirokikh, B., et al.: Universal loss reweighting to balance lesion size inequality in 3D medical image segmentation. In: Martel, A.L., et al. (eds.) MICCAI 2020. LNCS, vol. 12264, pp. 523–532. Springer, Cham (2020). https://doi.org/10.1007/978-3-030-59719-1_51

22. Wang, W., Chen, C., Ding, M., Yu, H., Zha, S., Li, J.: TransBTS: multimodal brain tumor segmentation using transformer. In: Bruijne, M., et al. (eds.) MICCAI 2021. LNCS, vol. 12901, pp. 109–119. Springer, Cham (2021). https://doi.org/10.1007/978-3-030-87193-2_11

23. Zhou, H.Y., et al.: nnFormer: volumetric medical image segmentation via a 3D Transformer. IEEE Trans. Image Process. 32, 4036–4045 (2023), https://github.com/282857341/nnFormer

24. Zhou, Z., Rahman Siddiquee, M.M., Tajbakhsh, N., Liang, J.: UNet++: a nested U-Net architecture for medical image segmentation. In: Stoyanov, D., et al. (eds.) DLMIA/ML-CDS -2018. LNCS, vol. 11045, pp. 3–11. Springer, Cham (2018). https://doi.org/10.1007/978-3-030-00889-5_1

25. Zhu, L.L., Lindenberg, R., Alexander, M.P., Schlaug, G.: Lesion load of the corticospinal tract predicts motor impairment in chronic stroke. Stroke **41**(5), 910–915 (2010)

# Virtual DSA for Learning Contrast Agent Dynamics in Projection Space

Noah Maul[1,2]([✉]), Annette Birkhold[2], Mareike Thies[1], Nastassia Vysotskaya[1], Fabian Wagner[1], Laura Pfaff[1], Markus Kowarschik[2], and Andreas Maier[1]

[1] Pattern Recognition Lab, Friedrich-Alexander Universitaet, Erlangen, Germany

[2] Siemens Healthineers AG, Forchheim, Germany
noah.maul@fau.de

**Abstract.** Digital Subtraction Angiography (DSA) is a well-established imaging modality supporting treatment and diagnosis of vascular pathologies. Various clinical DSA acquisition protocols exist that provide qualitative blood flow information for vascular diseases. Velocity quantification algorithms primarily rely on tracking a contrast agent (CA) bolus through the vasculature. However, the true CA velocity is fast compared to the frame rate of angiographic images. Therefore, high blood velocities pose a challenge for these methods, as the bolus may flow through long vessel segments between two subsequent DSA frames. This problem can be mitigated by increasing the temporal resolution, or equivalently, the projection image frame rate. We propose a simulation-informed neural network approach to synthetically double the projection frame rate without additional patient dose. We evaluate the quality of the synthesized projection images and show the impact on bolus tracking algorithms. Synthesized projection images can be predicted with a mean absolute percentage error of $2.5 \pm 0.8\,\%$ in the inflow phase. Further, the synthesized projections qualitatively capture bolus dynamics more accurately compared to linear interpolation. Conceptually, our method allows extension to predicting multiple intermediate projection frames, which can be a valuable tool toward accurate quantitative vascular flow estimation.

**Keywords:** Digital Subtraction Angiography · Computational Fluid Dynamics · Deep Learning · Cerebrovascular Blood Flow

## 1 Introduction

Diagnosis and treatment of vascular pathologies, such as aneurysms or stenoses, rely on fast and reliable estimation of hemodynamic information. During interventional procedures, hemodynamic information can be inferred from Digital Subtraction Angiography (DSA), which is an established x-ray-based imaging method for the visualization of blood vessels. The simplest form of DSA comprises a temporal sequence of single-view x-ray projections (2D-DSA), enabling

© The Author(s), under exclusive license to Springer Nature Switzerland AG 2025
R. Su et al. (Eds.): ISLES 2024/SWITCH 2024, LNCS 15408, pp. 51–60, 2025.
https://doi.org/10.1007/978-3-031-81101-2_6

blood dynamics visualization. Performing multi-view rotational acquisitions allows for additional static 3D reconstruction of the vasculature (3D-DSA). Current research [1,6,12] has focused on 4D-DSA reconstruction algorithms that enable qualitative flow visualization in 3D space. However, clinical decision making benefits from hemodynamic quantities, such as velocity or pressure values that are derived from the acquired data.

Several algorithms [9,13,14,17,18] have been proposed to estimate blood flow based on DSA images. In many cases, the algorithms rely on the tracking of the contrast agent (CA) bolus. Due to the cardiac cycle pulsatility, the injection of CA into the bloodstream leads to time-varying CA concentrations, resulting in measurable wave patterns. These CA waves are advected through the vasculature and can be spatially and temporally tracked to estimate velocities [14]. However, velocity estimation accuracy is strongly limited by temporal resolution that is equivalent to the frame rate at which projection images are recorded. Assuming a blood velocity of $1\,\mathrm{m\,s^{-1}}$ and a commonly used frame rate of 30 frames per second, the CA bolus is advected approximately $3.33\,\mathrm{cm}$, potentially flowing through multiple vessel segments between two frames. Hence, determining the contribution of velocities within the vessel segments to the total advected distance is not straightforward at this temporal resolution. However, an increased frame rate requires higher patient dose and faster detector readouts, posing technical challenges.

In this paper, our goal is to synthetically increase temporal resolution by utilizing knowledge about the fluid dynamics of blood and CA. For this purpose, we present a machine-learning-based method to estimate CA dynamics in projection space. The model is trained on a large dataset of virtual angiographic projection images based on high-resolution computational fluid dynamics (CFD) simulations. By training in a supervised manner on the synthetic data, we inform the network about underlying blood and CA dynamics, enabling the estimation of non-recorded projection images. Our pipeline consists of several steps: In a first step, we simulate the physiological blood flow, injection, and transport of CA in the cerebral vasculature. Second, a rotational DSA acquisition process is simulated and virtual projection images are computed. In a third step, we train a convolutional neural network (CNN) to predict the intermediate image between two projection images acquired at 30 frames per second. Repeated for the entire projection images sequence, the temporal resolution can be increased to 60 frames per second. We evaluate the quality of the interpolated projection images, as well as analyze the influence of the increased frame rate on bolus tracking.

## 2  Method

### 2.1  Problem Description and Overview

A 4D-DSA flow quantification task can be described as an inverse problem, where a time series of 2D x-ray projection images $\mathbf{Y} = (\mathbf{Y}_{t_1}, \ldots, \mathbf{Y}_{t_T} \mid \mathbf{Y}_{t_i} \in \mathbb{R}^{H_y \times W_y})$ is utilized to recover information about the time-dependent velocity

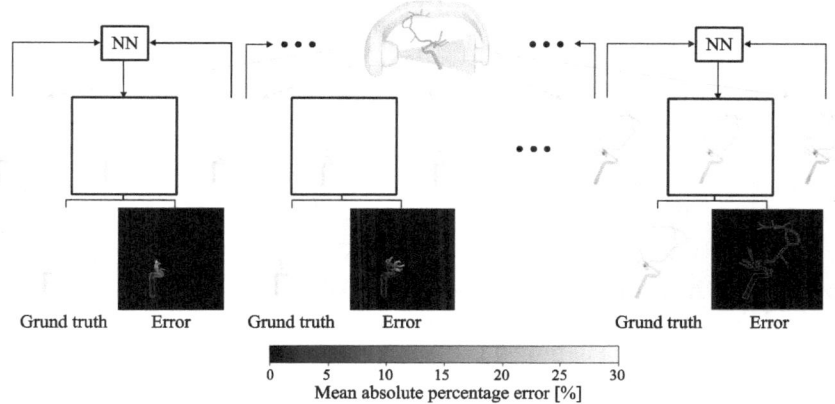

**Fig. 1.** Visualization of an exemplary trajectory from the test set. The neural network (NN) is iteratively applied to the whole sequence, estimating the inter-frame CA dynamics. Ground truth and error maps are depicted for each estimated projection. Erroneous regions are mainly limited to inflow regions with low CA concentration and therefore low x-ray attenuation

field $\mathbf{U}^{4D} = (\mathbf{U}^{3D}_{t_1}, \ldots, \mathbf{U}^{3D}_{t_T} \mid \mathbf{U}^{3D}_{t_i} \in \mathbb{R}^{H_x \times W_x \times D_x})$. After CA injection and mixture, the CA is distributed by the flow, leading to time-dependent 3D CA concentrations $\mathbf{X}^{4D} = (\mathbf{X}^{3D}_{t_1}, \ldots, \mathbf{X}^{3D}_{t_T} \mid \mathbf{X}^{3D}_{t_i} \in \mathbb{R}^{H_x \times W_x \times D_x})$ that are not directly observable. However, the filling states are connected to the projection images on the rotational trajectory through a cone-beam CT forward projection operator $A_{t_i}$

$$\mathbf{Y}_{t_i} = A_{t_i}(\mathbf{X}^{3D}_{t_i}) + \epsilon_{t_i}, \tag{1}$$

and a noise term $\epsilon_{t_i}$. In practice, only a discrete number of $T$ projection images are available, representing the temporal sampling points. However, the filling states $\mathbf{X}^{4D}$ and thus the projection images $\mathbf{Y}$ are temporally linked by a dynamic process governed by the laws of fluid mechanics. Assuming a continuous function $c : \mathbb{R}^4 \to \mathbb{R}$, providing the true CA concentration at each spatiotemporal point, and velocity field $\mathbf{u} : \mathbb{R}^4 \to \mathbb{R}^3$, the temporal dynamics can be described by a partial differential equation (PDE)

$$\frac{\partial c}{\partial t} = f(c, \mathbf{u}, \frac{\partial c}{\partial x}, \ldots). \tag{2}$$

In this work, we aim to directly estimate the contrast agent dynamics in projection space utilizing a neural network. In particular, we approximate the inter-frame dynamics $\mathbf{Y}_{t_{i+1}} = \mathbf{Y}_{t_i} + \int_{t_i}^{t_{i+1}} \frac{\partial A(c(\mathbf{x},t))}{\partial t} dt$ by feeding pairs of subsequent projection images acquired at 30 frames per second to the network. The network is trained to estimate the respective temporally intermediate state. For this purpose, approximately $260,000$ projection images are generated based on CFD simulations. Figure 1 exemplary depicts a sequence of projection images and highlights the iterative application of the network.

## 2.2 Virtual DSA Simulation and Dataset Generation

The neural network training requires a dataset of virtual DSA projection image sequences. We follow the pipeline of Maul et al. [10] to create a dataset based on cerebrovascular geometries from the AneuX dataset [7] and in-house surface meshes, which were all segmented from 3D rotational angiography reconstructions. In the following, we summarize each step in the pipeline and refer to the aforementioned study for details.

**Blood and CA Model.** We model blood and CA as a Newtonian incompressible fluid with a kinematic viscosity $\nu$ of $3.2 \times 10^{-6}\,\mathrm{m^2\,s^{-1}}$ and density of $1060\,\mathrm{kg\,m^{-3}}$. The flow is assumed to be laminar and can be described with the incompressible Navier-Stokes equations

$$\frac{\partial \mathbf{u}}{\partial t} + \mathbf{u} \cdot \nabla \mathbf{u} = -\nabla p + \nu \nabla^2 \mathbf{u}$$
$$\nabla \cdot \dot{\mathbf{u}} = 0 , \tag{3}$$

where $p$ denotes pressure. Further, vessel walls are modeled as rigid, with zero-gradient pressure and no-slip velocity boundary conditions (BCs). In order to simulate CA concentration maps, the blood flow model is coupled with a CA injection and transport model. In line with existing research [2–4,15,17], the mixture of CA and blood is modeled as a single-phase flow, however the velocity is influenced by CA injection. The CA transport can be described by an advection-diffusion equation of the CA concentration $c$

$$\frac{\partial c}{\partial t} = D\nabla^2 c - \mathbf{u} \cdot \nabla c , \tag{4}$$

where $D$ refers to a constant diffusion coefficient and $\mathbf{u}$ to the underlying velocity field. The CA is injected into the internal carotid artery (ICA) upstream the simulated domain and assumed to be fully mixed with blood at the inlet.

**X-Ray Simulation.** In a clinical setting, DSA projection images are acquired by subtracting a mask run (without CA injection) from a fill run (imaged during CA injection), which allows visualizing contrasted vessels only. The x-ray attenuation after subtraction is hence only caused by the blood CA mixture. As the x-ray attenuation of iodine-based CA is significantly higher than of blood, we perform a single-material cone beam forward projection to simulate the DSA protocol. The attenuation of the x-rays follows the Lambert-Beer law

$$\mathbf{Y}_{t_i}(\mathbf{v}) = \int I_0(E) \cdot \exp\left(-\mu(E) \int c(x,t)\,\mathrm{d}l\right) \mathrm{d}E , \tag{5}$$

where $\mathbf{Y}_{t_i}(\mathbf{v})$ is the intensity at detector pixel $\mathbf{v}$ and $I_0(E)$ the incident intensity for a given energy $E$ [16]. The linear attenuation coefficient of the CA $\mu = (\mu/\rho)_{\mathrm{CA}} \cdot \rho_{\mathrm{CA}}$ is the product of the mass attenuation coefficient $(\mu/\rho)_{\mathrm{CA}}$

and the CA density $\rho_{CA}$. The DSA images are simulated using the DeepDRR framework [16] using $(\mu/\rho)_{CA}$ of the *Ultravist-300* (Bayer Vital GmbH, Leverkusen, Germany) CA with an iopromide concentration of $623\,\mathrm{mg\,mL^{-1}}$.

**Dataset Generation.** We augment our dataset by simulating each vascular geometry with four different BCs and nine different x-ray geometry parameters (i.e., nine different circular trajectories). The physiological velocity inlet waveform is sampled from a reported distribution that is parameterized by three numbers: mean flow rate, cardiac cycle length, and age. We sample from the normal distributed mean flow rates and cardiac cycle lengths with the reported means and standard deviations. The age is chosen uniformly as either young or elderly [5]. For each BC, we generate nine different projection series by varying the starting primary angles $\alpha \in \{0°, 55°, 110°\}$ and secondary angles $\beta \in \{-20°, 0°, 20°\}$ to simulate varying head poses and augment our dataset. The simulation of different c-arm trajectories further increases our dataset size without running expensive CFD simulations and can be regarded as the simulation of varying head poses. The primary angle is increased by $0.85°$ for each timestep and 60 projection images per second are simulated.

### 2.3 Neural Network Model

Given a temporal sequence of projection images $\mathbf{Y} = (\mathbf{Y}_{t_1}, \ldots, \mathbf{Y}_{t_T} \mid \mathbf{Y}_{t_i} \in \mathbb{R}^{H_y \times W_y})$, we aim to approximate the inter-image CA dynamics. Instead of estimating the full dynamics between frames, we focus on estimating the intermediate projection $\mathbf{Y}_{t_{i+0.5}}$ between two subsequent frames $\mathbf{Y}_{t_i}$ and $\mathbf{Y}_{t_{i+1}}$. This approach acts as a data augmentation strategy, as several projection pairs can be extracted from each c-arm trajectory. Hence, we optimize our network to learn the mapping $(\mathbf{Y}_{t_i}, \mathbf{Y}_{t_{i+1}}) \rightarrow \mathbf{Y}_{t_{i+0.5}}$ for all possible pairs in the training set.

**Input Preprocessing.** We convert the projection images $\mathbf{Y}_{t_i}$ and $\mathbf{Y}_{t_{i+1}}$ to line integral domain by dividing the detector signal by the incident intensity $I_0$ and applying the negative logarithm. During training, we add random rotation, as well as horizontal and vertical flipping as augmentation techniques, since the flow is invariant to these transformations. We concatenate the two projection images, resulting in an input tensor with two channels.

**Network Architecture.** We utilize the exact original U-Net architecture proposed by Ronneberger et al. [11] for our neural network. The two-channel input tensor is fed to the network, processed and the estimated projection image is returned. During inference, we apply the network iteratively on the whole projection image time series.

**Dataset Split and Training.** We perform a patient-wise data split to avoid overlapping geometries between train, validation, and test set. Hence, we split the data into 35 train, 5 validation and 6 test geometries, resulting in 194 742, 30 546, and 36 063 projection images, respectively. The network is trained to minimize the mean absolute error $||\mathbf{Y}_{t_{i+0.5}} - \hat{\mathbf{Y}}_{t_{i+0.5}}||_1$ between ground truth $\mathbf{Y}_{t_{i+0.5}}$ and prediction $\hat{\mathbf{Y}}_{t_{i+0.5}}$. The background pixels outside the vessel tree are masked out in the loss calculation. We employ the Adam optimizer [8] with a batch size of 32 and a learning rate of $5 \times 10^{-3}$. The network is trained until validation loss convergence. We choose the model parameters corresponding to the lowest validation loss for evaluation.

## 3    Experiments and Results

### 3.1    Global Evaluation

To evaluate the overall performance of our model on the test set, we calculate statistics across all predicted projections that belong to the inflow phase ($\leq 0.5\,s$). The inflow phase is the time frame in which the vascular tree gets filled with CA and in which the bolus is most visible. Therefore, an accurate estimation is desired for bolus position estimation. We mask out pixel values $\leq 0.025$ to avoid averaging effects on the background, division by small numbers, and the influence of the slight spatial shift of the vessels due to increasing projection angle. We calculate the mean absolute percentage error between predicted $\hat{\mathbf{Y}}_{t_{i+0.5}}$ and ground truth projection image $\mathbf{Y}_{t_{i+0.5}}$ for pairs in the test set, and calculate mean, median, and standard deviation across the per-sample results. We visualize the error distribution in Fig. 2 and compare it to linear temporal interpolation. The global mean, median, and standard deviation of the percentage error across the set are 2.5%, 2.3%, and 0.8% for the network prediction and 5.6%, 4.6%, and 2.7% for linear interpolation.

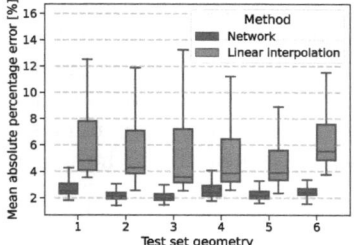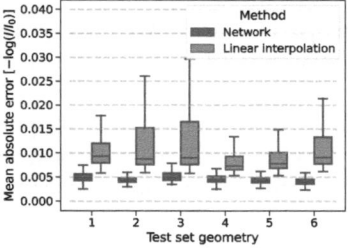

**Fig. 2.** Error distributions of the predicted inflow phase calculated individually for each vascular geometry in the test set. Most of the predicted projection images show a relative error smaller than 4%. Linear interpolation between two subsequent frames, however, leads to substantially higher errors. Outliers are excluded for improved visualization

## 3.2   Qualitative Projection Evaluation

For qualitative evaluation, we plot a subset of projection images from an exemplary trajectory from the test set in Fig. 1. It shows two predicted frames at the inflow stage and one frame with a filled vessel tree. We observe that there is a strong agreement between predicted and ground truth projection images. Erroneous regions are mainly limited to inflow regions with low CA concentration and therefore low x-ray attenuation. The projection image corresponding to the filled state can be predicted with high accuracy throughout the vasculature.

## 3.3   Qualitative Bolus Tracking Evaluation

DSA projection images can be utilized for hemodynamic estimation algorithms [14], where the exact spatiotemporal dynamics of the bolus is crucial to obtain accurate velocity estimates. We evaluate the bolus dynamics by qualitatively comparing the bolus transport in images based on linear and network interpolation. For this, we randomly select two geometries from the test set and pick a simulation with an average inflow rate of $5.3\,\mathrm{m\,L\,s^{-1}}$ and $6.6\,\mathrm{m\,L\,s^{-1}}$, respectively. Subsequently, inflow phase projections are compared and the bolus edge is highlighted. The results are visualized in Fig. 3. It can be observed that linearly interpolated frames tend to overestimate bolus advection.

# 4   Discussion

Inferring flow information from DSA projection images is an inverse problem, for which temporal resolution plays a crucial role. Due to high blood velocities in the main cerebral arteries, CA may be advected through several vessel segments between two measured x-ray projections. This poses a challenge to flow quantification methods, e.g., distance-density curve shift velocity estimation algorithms [14]. In this work, we train a neural network to learn the CA propagation dynamics in projection space, effectively doubling the temporal resolution synthetically. We inform the network about the underlying fluid dynamics of blood and CA by training it on a large dataset of artificial DSA acquisitions. We evaluate our method on the projection generation task, resulting in a mean absolute percentage error of $2.5 \pm 0.8\,\%$ between the simulated ground truth and prediction. Additionally, we analyze the influence of our method on bolus tracking and compare it to linear interpolation. Our method has some limitations. The simulation of the virtual DSA sequences requires substantial computational resources due to computationally expensive CFD simulations. However, multiple virtual c-arm trajectories and corresponding projection images can be generated per CFD simulation to augment the data set, increasing its size by an order of magnitude. Further, the application of our method to real clinical projection images requires further investigation. In this regard, domain adaptation methods may be useful to narrow the gap between simulated and real DSA projection images. In general, our method is conceptually not limited to predicting single intermediate projection images, as simulations enable the computation of virtual x-ray

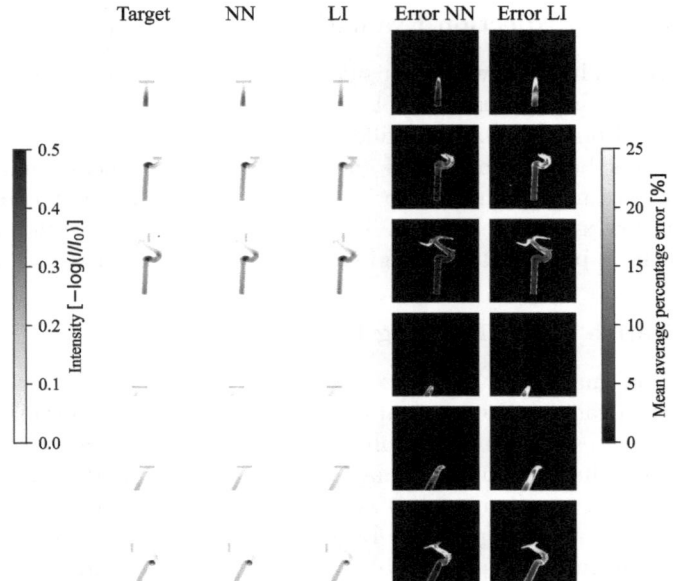

**Fig. 3.** Comparison of neural network (NN) and linearly interpolated (LI) projections for two sequences. The top three rows show projections of the first and the bottom rows projections of the second case. The NN-based interpolation accurately tracks the bolus, whereas LI tends to overestimate the intermediate advection between two recorded frames

images at any point in time. Hence, our method could be extended to estimate multiple intermediate frames between two acquired projections.

## 5    Conclusion

In conclusion, inferring flow information from DSA projection images is a challenging task that benefits from an increased temporal resolution. Our presented method is based on training a neural network on a dataset of virtual DSA acquisitions generated from high-resolution CFD simulations. The approach synthetically doubles the temporal resolution by predicting the intermediate frame between two adjacent projections. Our approach demonstrates promising performance and underscores the potential of the synergy of computational models and machine learning.

**Acknowledgments.** This project uses data from the AneuX morphology database, an open-access, multi-centric database combining data from three European projects: AneuX project (www.aneux.ch; @neurIST protocol v5; ethics autorisations Geneva BASEC PB_2018-00073; supported by the grant from the Swiss SystemsX.ch initiative, evaluated by the Swiss National Science Foundation),

@neurIST project (www.aneurist.org; @neurIST protocol v1; ethics autorisations Amsterdam MEC 07-159, Barcelona2007-3507, Geneva CER 07-056, Oxfordshire REC AQ05/Q1604/162, Pècs RREC MC P 06 Jul 2007; supported by the 6th framework program of the European Commission FP6-IST-2004-027703) and Aneurisk (http://ecm2.mathcs.emory.edu/aneuriskweb/index). The work of Fabian Wagner, Mareike Thies, and Andreas Maier was supported by the European Research Council (ERC) under the European Union's Horizon 2020 research and innovation program (ERC Grant No. 810316).

**Disclosure of Interests.** The authors have no competing interests to declare that are relevant to the content of this article.

**Disclaimer.** The concepts and information presented are based on research and are not commercially available.

# References

1. Davis, B., et al.: 4D digital subtraction angiography: implementation and demonstration of feasibility. Am. J. Neuroradiol. **34**, 1914–1921 (2013)
2. Durant, J., Waechter, I., Hermans, R., Weese, J., Aach, T.: Toward quantitative virtual angiography: Evaluation with in vitro studies. In: 2008 5th IEEE International Symposium on Biomedical Imaging: From Nano to Macro, pp. 632–635 (2008)
3. Endres, J., et al.: A workflow for patient-individualized virtual angiogram generation based on CFD simulation. Comput. Math. Methods Med. **2012**, 1–24 (2012)
4. Ford, M.D., et al.: Virtual angiography for visualization and validation of computational models of aneurysm hemodynamics. IEEE Trans. Med. Imaging **24**(12), 1586–1592 (2005)
5. Hoi, Y., et al.: Characterization of volumetric flow rate waveforms at the carotid bifurcations of older adults. Physiol. Measurem. **31**, 291–302 (2010)
6. Huizinga, N., Keil, F., Birkhold, A., Kowarschik, M., Tritt, S., Berkefeld, J.: 4D flat panel conebeam CTA for in vivo imaging of the microvasculature of the human cortex with a novel software prototype. Am. J. Neuroradiol. **41**, 976–979 (2020)
7. Juchler, N., Schilling, S., Bijlenga, P., Kurtcuoglu, V., Hirsch, S.: Shape trumps size: image-based morphological analysis reveals that the 3D shape discriminates intracranial aneurysm disease status better than aneurysm size. Front. Neurol. **13** (2022)
8. Kingma, D.P., Ba, J.: Adam: a method for stochastic optimization. In: 3rd International Conference on Learning Representations, ICLR (2015)
9. Maul, N., et al.: Transient hemodynamics prediction using an efficient octree-based deep learning model. In: Information Processing in Medical Imaging, pp. 183–194. Springer Nature Switzerland, Cham (2023). https://doi.org/10.1007/978-3-031-34048-2_15
10. Maul, N., et al.: Physics-Informed Learning for Time-Resolved Angiographic Contrast Agent Concentration Reconstruction. arXiv preprint arXiv:2403.01993 (2024)
11. Ronneberger, O., Fischer, P., Brox, T.: U-Net: convolutional networks for biomedical image segmentation. In: Navab, N., Hornegger, J., Wells, W.M., Frangi, A.F. (eds.) MICCAI 2015. LNCS, vol. 9351, pp. 234–241. Springer, Cham (2015). https://doi.org/10.1007/978-3-319-24574-4_28

12. Ruedinger, K., Schafer, S., Speidel, M., Strother, C.: 4D-DSA: development and current neurovascular applications. Am. J. Neuroradiol. **42**, 214–220 (2021)
13. Shaughnessy, G., Schafer, S., Speidel, M.A., Strother, C.M., Mistretta, C.A.: Measuring blood velocity using 4D-DSA: a feasibility study. Med. Phys. **45**, 4510–4518 (2018)
14. Shpilfoygel, S.D., Close, R.A., Valentino, D.J., Duckwiler, G.R.: X-ray videodensitometric methods for blood flow and velocity measurement: a critical review of literature. Med. Phys. **27**, 2008–2023 (2000)
15. Sun, Q., Groth, A., Aach, T.: Comprehensive validation of computational fluid dynamics simulations of in-vivo blood flow in patient-specific cerebral aneurysms. Med. Phys. **39**, 742–754 (2012)
16. Unberath, M., et al.: DeepDRR – a catalyst for machine learning in fluoroscopy-guided procedures. In: Frangi, A.F., Schnabel, J.A., Davatzikos, C., Alberola-López, C., Fichtinger, G. (eds.) MICCAI 2018. LNCS, vol. 11073, pp. 98–106. Springer, Cham (2018). https://doi.org/10.1007/978-3-030-00937-3_12
17. Waechter, I., Bredno, J., Hermans, R., Weese, J., Barratt, D.C., Hawkes, D.J.: Model-based blood flow quantification from rotational angiography. Med. Image Anal. **12**, 586–602 (2008)
18. Wu, Y., et al.: Quantification of blood velocity with 4D digital subtraction angiography using the shifted least-squares method. Am. J. Neuroradiol. **39**, 1871–1877 (2018)

# Robust Feature Selection for Classifying Early Ischemic Changes in Posterior Stroke

Leonhard Rist[1,2]($\boxtimes$), Hendrik Ditt[2], Michael Sühling[2], Valentin Honus[3], Peter Schramm[3], Andreas Maier[1], and Oliver Taubmann[2]

[1] Friedrich-Alexander-Universität Erlangen-Nürnberg, Erlangen, Germany
leonhard.rist@fau.de
[2] CT R&D Image Analytics, Siemens Healthineers, Forchheim, Germany
[3] Radiology and Neuroradiology, University Hospital Schleswig-Holstein, Lübeck, Germany

**Abstract.** Fast assessment in stroke diagnosis is essential to improve the treatment outcome. Scoring systems such as the ASPECT score facilitate the triage of patients according to stroke severity. For occlusions in the posterior circulation, pcASPECTS evaluates whether certain posterior cerebral regions show early signs of stroke and can be applied using the admission NCCT scan. This work investigates the automatic classification of early stroke changes in the two largest posterior regions based on NCCT images. The main focus lies on the implementation of robust measures that can counteract noise and scanner variances since they are harmful to established Radiomics pipelines. For 170 respectively derived regions from 85 patients, the described pipeline can reach up to 83.84% AUC with 79.40% sensitivity for the cerebellum and 73.14% AUC with 57.97% sensitivity for the occipital regions. A simple in-patient normalization scheme proved to be the most effective measure by improving the AUC by +8.17% and the sensitivity by +16.80%. Additional robustness techniques such as noise augmentation or discarding unstable and correlated features using the post-treatment scan resulted in only slight deviations from the best result, making them valuable tools for improving robustness when using Radiomics for posterior stroke classification.

## 1 Introduction

Ischemic stroke outcome benefits highly from fast assessment and short therapy times [7,18]. Otherwise, the limited blood and oxygen flow leads an increasing number of dying cerebral cells which can result in subtle to distinct changes of the parenchyma in the routinely acquired initial non-contrast computed tomography (NCCT) scan. The treatment decision towards thrombolysis and/or mechanical thrombectomy depends upon the location of the occlusion (visible in CT angiography imaging), onset time and volume of affected brain areas. For easier communication and fast rule-based decision-making for triage, predefined scores such as the ASPECTS (Alberta Stroke Program Early CT Score) [1,17] and pcASPECTS (posterior circulation) [15] exist, counting the affected regions. ASPECTS defines 10 symmetric regions supplied by the arteria media and can be evaluated by comparing the intensity of each region with its hemispherical counterpart. Automatic ASPECTS evaluation tools compute the score based on asymmetric features between the hemispheres, showing good agreement with neuroradiologist readings [13,19]. However, posterior circulation regions require more involved assessment techniques. The posterior regions consist of the left-right symmetrical cerebellum, occipital and smaller thalamus regions as well as the individual pons and midbrain sections in the brain stem. In contrast to what is typically seen in the (media-supplied) ASPECTS regions, the symmetric posterior regions can be affected either individually or jointly. Additionally, the non-symmetric regions do not have a counterpart for comparison. Hence, an automatic evaluation cannot rely on simple intensity differences and requires sophisticated feature extraction to build trainable models. These were also proposed for ASPECT scoring, either using Radiomics features [11] or deep-asymmetry convolutional networks [2].

However, the complexity of the task coupled with data scarcity of labeled early posterior stroke changes renders state-of-the-art convolutional neural networks infeasible. To decrease the dimensionality of such problems, predefined Radiomics (first-order image and texture) features with smart feature selection have proven to reliably solve many medical classification tasks [12] when using classical machine learning models. For the pcASPECTS regions, Kniep et al. [9,10] were the first to investigate the use of Radiomics in early ischemic changes using a Random Forest classifier, exhibiting performance on equal terms or even surpassing human readers. However, since such features are affected by scanner differences and noise patterns, robustness is a major concern of such approaches [16]. Various approaches in the field of Radiomics exist to counteract these problems while the clinical workflow of the problem itself also holds potential for better homogenization of the processed NCCT scans.

This work demonstrates the integration of existing and new principles adapted to tools available in the stroke workflow, aiming to increase robustness during feature selection for region-wise early onset change classification in NCCT. We investigate the two biggest symmetrical regions relevant for pcASPECTS, shown in Fig. 1 leaving out regions in the brain stem. On one hand, due to lower image quality, on the other hand because changes in brain stem already indicate severe stroke or long onset times, resulting in few to no treatment options. Presented methods include the exploitation of unaffected regions of the acute NCCT scans for an in-patient normalization scheme and noise estimation for augmentation. Additionally, we make use of the post-treatment scan during the feature selection step to rule out uncorrelated features. Finally, we thoroughly investigate all parts of the training pipeline to give guidelines for each step, ranging from the choice of reconstructed slice thickness, use of oversampling techniques and number of features, to the choice of the underlying model. All experiments are carried out on a heterogeneous dataset from multiple scanners consisting of 85 patients (170 samples each for cerebellum and occipital region).

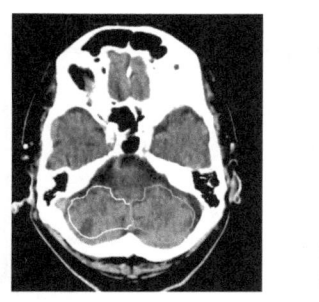 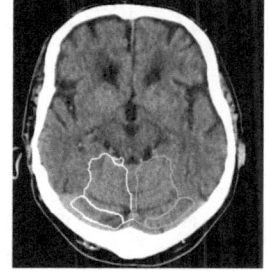 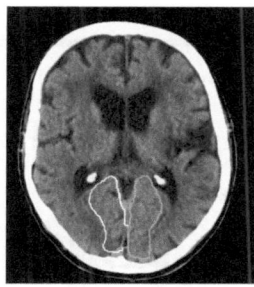

(a) Cerebellum          (b) Cerebellum & occipital          (c) Occipital regions

**Fig. 1.** Example NCCT scan with registered left and right cerebellum and occipital regions. Affected regions are red, healthy regions green. (Color figure online)

## 2    Materials and Methods

### 2.1    Data

The data used in this work stems from a retrospective study (Institutional Review Board approval, need for informed consent was waived) of 85 patients with posterior ischemic stroke who were all treated using thrombectomy. Each patient sample contains the acute NCCT scan with 1 and 5 mm slice thickness. Additionally, post-intervention scans are also available as thin- and thick slice images. For each patient, the region-wise classification according to pcASPECTS is available. The reading was performed by a highly experienced neuroradiologist using only the acute 5 mm images. Of the respective 170 regions used for training and testing, 27 cerebellum regions were affected, 15 on the left hemisphere and 12 on the right in total with an overlap on 9 patients. In the 31 affected occipital regions, 18 early changes were visible on the left side and 13 on the right side while the overlap among patients was smaller with a value of 6. The data was acquired with 4 different reconstruction kernels from two different vendors.

### 2.2    Data Extraction and Preprocessing

First, the relevant regions of the NCCT scan must be extracted. The different extraction steps are depicted in the upper row of Fig. 2. After the acquisition, we non-rigidly register a three-dimensional brain atlas [8] to the NCCT scan. This atlas was extended by incorporating the sub-regions of all ASPECTS and pcASPECTS regions from which we select the cerebellum and occipital regions for further processing. Regions of bone are excluded from the extraction to get a more homogeneous distribution.

The data was collected from different scanners and additionally reconstructed with different kernels, which show dissimilar intensity offsets and characteristics, see Fig. 3a, and hence require data normalization. Using the standard deviation and intensity mean of the M1-M6 ASPECTS regions, we can apply an in-patient

# Data preparation

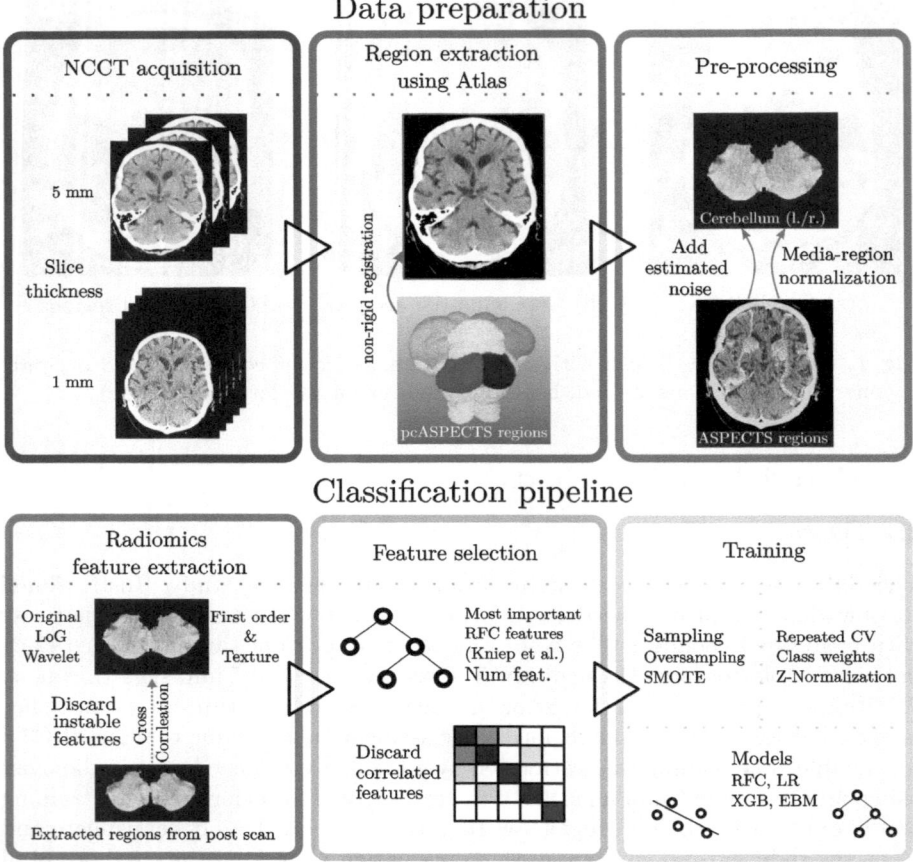

**Fig. 2.** Pipeline for data extraction, feature selection and classification. Investigated parameters are highlighted in green. (Color figure online)

z-normalization of the extracted cerebellum and occipital regions, leveling the intensities across different configurations, see Fig. 3b.

Noise is an important factor in CT imaging in general and specifically when applying Radiomics features. As proposed by GÃűtz et al. [6], we apply DAFIT by adding additional Gaussian noise to the scans before feature extraction. This is done twice, doubling the available data with the intention to make the feature selection process independent of noise. To estimate realistic standard deviations of the simulated noise, we again make use of the ASPECTS regions as they contain small homogeneous areas and use the region with the lowest variance for noise characteristics estimation. Both of these intra-scan robustness methods for normalization across scanners and augmentation are fully automatic and do not require additional imaging.

## 2.3   Feature Extraction and Classification

After extraction of the 4 respective regions, the 3D volumes are converted into scalar features to be processed by classical machine learning approaches. Each symmetric region pair is used to jointly train one estimator. Radiomics features are used as a well-established substitute for trainable feature extractors to derive global first-order and local texture features. Following Kniep et al. [10], all first-order and texture features (from the pyradiomics library [5]) are computed using the original, the Laplacian of Gaussians and the Wavelet image, resulting in 837 features. However, to build reliable machine learning models, the feature set should be reduced to contain only informative and stable features.

To further increase robustness, we make use of the post-treatment scan that is routinely acquired after therapeutic intervention. This scan is only necessary for the feature selection before model training, not for inference. Following the data preprocessing steps of the acute NCCT scan in Sect. 2.2, we extract the relevant regions from the post-scan. Features of a region unaffected by the acute stroke should be consistent between pre- and post-scan. Hence, one can calculate the cross-correlation coefficient of these samples in the training split and discard features if their respective correlation is below the threshold $t_1 < 0.8$ [6]. This feature – while possibly bearing information for the specific training set – cannot be considered robust. Next, we would like to reduce the feature space by only choosing relevant features. Following Kniep et al. [10], we fit a Random Forest Classifier (RFC) on all remaining features and select the most informative ones by using the Gini impurity metric. To further reduce redundancy in the selected features, we perform an additional correlation cluster analysis where only the most important features in a correlation cluster formed by absolute correlation values of $t_2 > 0.9$ are kept [6]. Finally, from this subgroup, only the $n$ most important features are used to train the final classifiers.

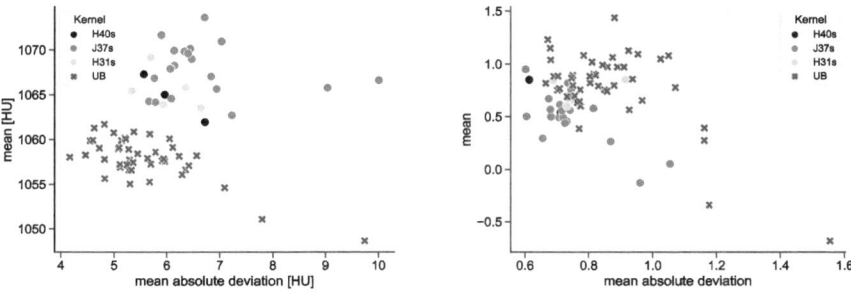

(a) Without in-patient normalization.     (b) With in-patient normalization

**Fig. 3.** Effect of different scanners and reconstruction kernels for the right cerebellum data. Exemplary values are intensity mean and the mean absolute deviation.

## 2.4   Experiments

We follow Kniep et al. [10] in their evaluation scheme, using a 5-fold cross-validation (CV) on 10 different random seeds and average the results. The data for the CV is stratified according to class labels and patients. Due to the limited amount of data and the CV evaluation scheme, we refrain from using iterative training methods that rely on another internal validation (tuning) set for parameter selection such as those used in neural networks. To give a broader picture of the performance of tabular data we compare multiple classifiers, specifically Random Forest Classifier (RFC), Linear Regression (LR), XGBoost [4] and Explainable Boosting Machines (EBM) [14]. All models are trained using inverse class frequency weighting. As evaluation metrics, we will mainly investigate the Area Under Receiver Operating Curve (AUC), balanced accuracy (B-Acc) and sensitivity.

As this work evaluates Radiomics feature robustness, we will provide an ablation study of the mentioned parameters in Sects. 2.2 and 2.3. All investigated parameters are also highlighted in green in Fig. 2. Namely, we will evaluate the impact of **slice thickness**, investigating whether using detailed but noisier 1 mm scans can be beneficial compared to the established 5 mm scans. To compensate for inter-scanner variances, we evaluate the proposed **in-patient normalization** scheme. Further, we will investigate the benefit of best-practice robustness methods adapted to our task, including **DAFIT augmentation** by adding noise before feature extraction and using **correlation** metrics for discarding unstable features using the post-treatment scans and via correlation cluster analysis. Also, typical data processing and model choices are investigated such as the **number of features** (5, 10 or 20), using **oversampling** techniques (none, random oversampling, SMOTE [3]) to counter class imbalance as well as using 4 increasingly complex **models** (LR, RFC, XGB, EMB). Note that without in-patient normalization, the selection of stable features via the post-scan yielded an insufficient amount of features for $n > 5$. Hence, $t_1$ was lowered to 0.7 for these cases to perform the experiments. Finally, the chosen feature groups of the selection process are also evaluated.

## 3   Results

This section first presents the best results (according to balanced accuracy) and configurations using Table 1, and afterwards discusses the ablation of all pipeline parts starting from the best model of the cerebellum using Table 2. Note that the averaged results are reported for the $10 \times$ repeated 5-fold CV.

*Model Selection and Best Configuration.* Overall, changes in the cerebellum were detected more reliably compared to the occipital regions by all models, most importantly with higher sensitivity. Our experiments show that for most configurations, Linear Regression with a small number of features is superior to more complex models, resulting in the best performing models for the cerebellum and occipital regions, see Table 1. The normalization within each patient and the 5 mm slice thickness were used for all the best models. For the cerebellum, all models were able to achieve performances between 74.06 - 83.84% AUC, however competitive sensitivity was only achievable with Linear Regression. Using the RFC resulted in the lowest standard deviations of the AUC. Using the SMOTE oversampling technique and a low number of features proved better for the cerebellum.

The best models for the occipital regions used more features, resulting in the top values of 68.3% B-Acc for the EBM and 73.14% AUC for the LR. It is noteworthy that different model architectures consistently struggled with different samples. For all regions, only Wavelet transformed features were selected when using $n=5$, mostly from the texture feature groups. Most prominently for the cerebellum, in 60% of the data splits the normalized gray-level non-uniformity was chosen (LLH and LHH filtered). The chosen features in the occipital case had a higher degree of low-pass filtering on average, mainly consisting of textural features. Informational Measure of Correlation (IMC) 2 and maximum probability (both LLL filtered) were the most prominent, chosen in 74 and 68% of the splits. The selected features are independent of the used models.

**Table 1.** Best model configurations. Metrics are given in %.

| Cerebellum | Thick. | Pat. norm | DAFIT | Corr. | # feat | Samp. | AUC | B-Acc | Sens. |
|---|---|---|---|---|---|---|---|---|---|
| Linear Reg | 5 | ✓ | ✗ | ✓ | 5 | SMOTE | **83.84** | 78.29 | **79.40** |
| RFC | 5 | ✓ | ✗ | ✗ | 20 | SMOTE | 77.11 | 71.47 | 54.87 |
| XGBoost | 5 | ✓ | ✓ | ✗ | 5 | SMOTE | 74.06 | 70.24 | 56.56 |
| EBM | 5 | ✓ | ✗ | ✗ | 5 | no | 74.92 | **80.14** | 61.73 |
| Occipital | Thick. | Pat. norm | DAFIT | Corr. | # feat | Samp. | AUC | B-Acc | Sens. |
| Linear Reg | 5 | ✓ | ✗ | ✗ | 5 | no | **73.14** | 67.47 | **57.97** |
| RFC | 5 | ✓ | ✗ | ✗ | 10 | Over | 62.05 | 63.55 | 39.10 |
| XGBoost | 5 | ✓ | ✓ | ✗ | 10 | SMOTE | 69.98 | 66.17 | 47.30 |
| EBM | 5 | ✓ | ✗ | ✗ | 10 | no | 65.71 | **68.30** | 51.19 |

*Data Preparation.* The reported ablation study for the best linear regression model in Table 2 reveals that the biggest positive influence on AUC, B-Acc and Sensitivity stems from the in-patient normalization technique, increasing the balanced accuracy by over 10%. Furthermore, with 1 mm slice thickness, the prediction performance only drops by 4.15% AUC even though being expected to be much less robust for Radiomics methods. Augmenting the scan with additive noise results in a small performance drop of 2% AUC while making the approach more robust against noise during feature selection.

*Feature Selection.* Not filtering for stable features using the post-treatment scan and dropping correlated feature clusters results in a negligible performance drop of 0.30% AUC, however the standard deviation across the runs and folds decreased without this measure by 2.35 %. Especially using more features increases this discrepancy between different data splits, along with a substantial decrease in sensitivity of over 10%.

**Table 2.** Ablation study. Results are presented relative to the values of the cerebellum linear regression model (Table 1). Values are in %, ± AUC indicates the standard deviation of the AUC.

| Parameter | Best | Ablation | AUC | ± AUC | B-Acc | Sens. | Spec. |
|---|---|---|---|---|---|---|---|
| Thickness | 5 | 1 mm | −4.15 | −0.86 | −5.86 | −6.27 | −5.43 |
| Patient-norm | ✓ | ✗ | −8.17 | +0.40 | −10.49 | −16.80 | −4.16 |
| DAFIT | ✗ | ✓ | −1.92 | +0.05 | −0.84 | −0.67 | −0.99 |
| Correlation | ✓ | ✗ | −0.30 | −2.34 | −1.35 | −1.20 | −1.47 |
| Num feat | 5 | 10 | −5.15 | +2.21 | −4.99 | −11.07 | +1.10 |
| Num feat | 5 | 20 | −6.67 | +3.00 | −3.79 | −10.07 | + 2.51 |

## 4   Discussion

This work presents a comprehensive pipeline for the detection of early ischemic changes in NCCT of patients with a posterior circulation stroke, namely in the cerebellum and occipital regions. Building on the work of Kniep et al. [10], we extend the proposed trainable Radiomics pipeline by various components to increase robustness. For this purpose, we utilize components that are inherent to the clinical workflow in stroke assessment during feature selection, such as other extracted regions from ASPECTS calculation for normalization and augmentation and the post-treatment scan for removing unstable features. The aspect of robustness is crucial in applied clinical routine when models are deployed on different scanners and sites, especially considering that the posterior part of the brain often exhibits lower image quality due to the high amount of surrounding bone. The best results were achieved with the model of lowest complexity (linear regression) and a low number of features (5). This hints that with the small amount of available data used, generalization can only be achieved by underfitting the data with low-variance models or by using strong regularization. More data is necessary to be able to exploit more complex patterns in the data.

Taking the difficulty of the task into account, the achieved AUC of almost 84% with a sensitivity close to 80% is in a competitive range for the cerebellum, also compared to the result of Kniep et al. [10] reporting 70% AUC with 60% sensitivity. Note, that the occipital regions perform worse in comparison with a maximal AUC of 73.14% (80% for Kniep et al.). However, the images in the comparison work were all acquired with the same dual-source CT scanner with standardized acquisition parameters (e.g. H30s reconstruction kernel), strengthening our proposed pipeline extension. The simple in-patient normalization is responsible for the highest influence on the performance, decreasing the variance of the intensity distribution of 4 different reconstruction kernels from two vendors to a more representative joint mean, see Fig. 3. Augmenting with additive noise before the feature extraction and discarding unstable and correlated features [6] only impacts the performance slightly. Here, the impact of noise was probably small due to mostly selected low-pass filtered features. Small performance differences for all of the mentioned methods due to ruling out potential information from the training set, are sufficiently compensated for by increased robustness.

For future work, tackling the problem with 3D convolutional neural networks in the volumetric domain could potentially exploit local patterns in a more direct way. Additionally, it gives the flexibility to predict multiple regions jointly, which would require for example a graph neural network layer in our scenario. However, initial CNN experiments were not able to generalize on the available data set.

## 5   Conclusion

This work investigates robustness measures for the classification of early ischemic changes in NCCT images of posterior stroke, e.g. for the application of pcASPECT scoring. In a dataset of 85 patients, 170 regions were extracted of the left-right symmetric cerebellum (27 cases affected) and occipital regions (31 affected). The described Radiomics pipeline can reach up to 83.84% AUC with 79.40% sensitivity for the cerebellum and 73.14% AUC with 57.97% sensitivity for the occipital regions. The most effective method to counter inter-scanner variances was a simple in-patient normalization scheme that had an effect of +8.17% on the AUC (+16.80% Sens.). Additional techniques such as noise augmentation, and discarding unstable and correlated features using the post-treatment scan, only resulted in slight deviations from the best result, making them valuable tools for improving robustness. Overall, we present a comprehensive set of measures to improve the prediction of early NCCT changes in posterior stroke scenarios which can be treated as a tool set when developing clinical applications in time-critical stroke decision-making.

## References

1. Cagnazzo, F., et al.: Mechanical thrombectomy in patients with acute ischemic stroke and aspects $< = 6$: a meta-analysis. J. NeuroInterventional Surg. **12**, 350–355 (2020). https://doi.org/10.1136/NEURINTSURG-2019-015237
2. Cao, Z., et al.: Deep learning derived automated aspects on nonâĂŘcontrast ct scans of acute ischemic stroke patients. Human Brain Mapp. **43**, 3023 (2022). https://doi.org/10.1002/HBM.25845
3. Chawla, N.V., Bowyer, K.W., Hall, L.O., Kegelmeyer, W.P.: Smote: synthetic minority over-sampling technique. J. Artif. Int. Res. **16**(1), 321–357 (2002)
4. Chen, T., Guestrin, C.: Xgboost: A scalable tree boosting system. In: Proceedings of the 22nd ACM SIGKDD International Conference on Knowledge Discovery and Data Mining, pp. 785–794. KDD '16, Association for Computing Machinery, New York, NY, USA (2016). https://doi.org/10.1145/2939672.2939785

5. Griethuysen, J.J.V., et al.: Computational radiomics system to decode the radiographic phenotype. Cancer Res. **77**, e104–e107 (2017). https://doi.org/10.1158/0008-5472.CAN-17-0339

6. Götz, M., Maier-Hein, K.H.: Optimal statistical incorporation of independent feature stability information into radiomics studies. Sci. Rep. 2020 10:1 **10**, 1–10 (2020). https://doi.org/10.1038/s41598-020-57739-8

7. Hacke, W., et al.: Association of outcome with early stroke treatment: pooled analysis of atlantis, ecass, and ninds rt-pa stroke trials. The Lancet **363**(9411), 768–774 (2004). https://doi.org/10.1016/S0140-6736(04)15692-4

8. Kemmling, A., Wersching, H., Berger, K., Knecht, S., Groden, C., Nölte, I.: Decomposing the hounsfield unit: probablistic segmentation of brain tissue in computed tomography. Clin. Neuroradiology 2011 22:1 **22**, 79–91 (2012). https://doi.org/10.1007/S00062-011-0123-0

9. Kniep, H.C., et al.: Imaging-based outcome prediction in posterior circulation stroke. J. Neurology **269**, 3800–3809 (2022)

10. Kniep, H.C., et al.: Posterior circulation stroke: machine learning-based detection of early ischemic changes in acute non-contrast ct scans. J. Neurology **267**, 2632–2641 (2020)

11. Kuang, H., et al.: Automated aspects on noncontrast ct scans in patients with acute ischemic stroke using machine learning. American Journal of Neuroradiology **40**, 33–38 (2019). https://doi.org/10.3174/AJNR.A5889

12. Lambin, P., et al.: Radiomics: the bridge between medical imaging and personalized medicine. Nature Rev. Clin. Oncol. 2017 14:12 **14**, 749–762 (2017). https://doi.org/10.1038/nrclinonc.2017.141

13. Li, L., et al.: Comparison of the performance between frontier aspects software and different levels of radiologists on assessing ct examinations of acute ischaemic stroke patients. Clin. Radiol. **75**(5), 358–365 (2020). https://doi.org/10.1016/j.crad.2019.12.010

14. Lou, Y., Caruana, R., Gehrke, J., Hooker, G.: Accurate intelligible models with pairwise interactions. In: Proceedings of the 19th ACM SIGKDD International Conference on Knowledge Discovery and Data Mining. p. 623-631. KDD '13, Association for Computing Machinery, New York, NY, USA (2013). https://doi.org/10.1145/2487575.2487579

15. Lu, W.Z., Lin, H.A., Bai, C.H., Lin, S.F.: Posterior circulation acute stroke prognosis early ct scores in predicting functional outcomes: a meta-analysis. PLoS ONE **16** (2021). https://doi.org/10.1371/JOURNAL.PONE.0246906

16. Mackin, D., et al.: Measuring ct scanner variability of radiomics features. Investigative radiology **50**, 757 (2015). https://doi.org/10.1097/RLI.0000000000000180

17. Pexman, J.H.W., et al.: Use of the alberta stroke program early ct score (aspects) for assessing ct scans in patients with acute stroke. Am. J. Neuroradiol. **22**, 1534–1542 (2001)

18. Saver, J.L.E.A.: Time to treatment with endovascular thrombectomy and outcomes from ischemic stroke: a meta-analysis. JAMA **316**(12), 1279–1289 (2016). https://doi.org/10.1001/jama.2016.13647, https://doi.org/10.1001/jama.2016.13647

19. Wolff, L., et al.: Validation of automated alberta stroke program early ct score (aspects) software for detection of early ischemic changes on non-contrast brain ct scans. Neuroradiology **63**, 491–498 (2021)

# ArterialGNet: Impossible Femoral Access Prediction in Stroke Mechanical Thrombectomy with Vascular Centerline Graph Embeddings

Pere Canals[1,2(✉)], Alvaro García-Tornel[1], and Marc Ribo[1,2]

[1] Stroke Unit, Neurology, Hospital Vall d'Hebron, Barcelona, Spain
pere.canals@vhir.org
[2] Departament de Medicina, Universitat Autònoma de Barcelona, Barcelona, Spain

**Abstract.** Extracranial vascular tortuosity is considered one of the most relevant factors leading to failed mechanical thrombectomy during stroke treatment. Currently, no objective method exists to reliably identify patients that will present difficulties or impossibility for cervical catheter access during endovascular interventions. Vascular tortuosity may be relevant at different scales, from general descriptors of a complete arterial pathway to local abnormalities which may introduce obstacles impossible to overcome during endovascular interventions. Arterial centerline maps have been widely used to characterize vascular tortuosity, and can be trivially represented as graphs. Graph neural networks offer unique properties that make them a great fit when dealing with these vascular descriptors. In this work, we present ArterialGNet, a graph neural network designed to integrate graph embeddings at multiple scales derived from vascular centerline pathways automatically extracted from CTA. A retrospective dataset comprised of 493 interventions with available CTA, including 19 (3.9%) where cervical access was impossible through transfemoral approach, was used for this study. Our model presents excellent discrimination ability ($AUROC = 0.89$, 95%CI, 0.88–0.90), outperforming previous approaches. Effective prediction of impossible femoral access may provide decision support to neurointerventionalists, leading to reduced procedural times and improved clinical outcomes in specific patients. Source code is available at https://github.com/perecanals/arterial_gnet.git.

**Keywords:** Stroke · CT · Thrombectomy · Geometric Learning · Attention Mechanism

## 1 Introduction

Endovascular thrombectomy has rapidly become the standard of care for patients with large vessel occlusion. Despite the high rates of treatment success of endovascular thrombectomy, with reperfusion rates over 90% in most recent trials [1], there is still room for improvement in selected cohorts. Impossible transfemoral catheter access remains one of the leading causes of unsuccessful reperfusion, accounting for up to a third of treatment failures [2, 3]. Although impossibility to reach the occlusion due to vessel tortuosity is rare (4.4%) [4], it has consistently been linked to decreased rates of reperfusion and poor clinical outcomes [5-11].

R. Su et al. (Eds.): ISLES 2024/SWITCH 2024, LNCS 15408, pp. 71–80, 2025.
https://doi.org/10.1007/978-3-031-81101-2_8

In recent years, the use of alternative access via the radial artery approach has surfaced as an effective strategy to address this challenge [12, 13]. Radial access seems to be non-inferior to femoral in terms of successful reperfusion rates and favorable functional outcomes, but it also may reduce the time from arterial puncture to thrombectomy initiation in selected cohort [12, 13]. However, transradial catheterization does not guarantee a fast access to the occlusion site and anatomical features may also be responsible of delays or impossible access.

Previous work that has studied the influence of tortuosity on difficult access or procedural duration has often relied on approaches that reduced tortuosity analysis to only a few features [10, 11, 14, 15]. Certain features encompass morphologies that involve multiple segments of the entire vascular anatomy (e.g., bovine aortic arch, aortic arch type), while others involve measurements taken on individual vascular segments (e.g., tortuosity index of the internal carotid artery), and still others concentrate on local morphology (e.g., presence of a kink along a centerline segment). It is crucial to acknowledge that tortuosity features affecting carotid catheterization may be significant at various levels of scale.

Arterial centerline maps (ACMs) have proven valuable in characterizing vascular tortuosity [16] and are make powerful descriptors of the vascular anatomy, while inherently forming connectivity networks that can be trivially represented by graphs. Furthermore, ACMs can encode information at various scales through adjustments in centerline sampling density, offering flexibility in feature computation while preserving connectivity.

Graph neural networks (GNNs) have demonstrated exceptional performance in vessel labeling tasks, leveraging ACMs and vascular segmentation 3D meshes [17-20]. GNNs possess unique capabilities that make them ideal for processing graphs derived from vascular ACMs, including the ability to handle variable-size inputs and encode features in both nodes and edges, all with minimal computational overhead.

In this study, we introduce ArterialGNet, a novel geometric learning model based on graph attention mechanisms that leverages tortuosity features extracted from ACMs at multiple scales and is trained to predict the feasibility of transfemoral catheter access on an individual patient basis during endovascular thrombectomy. This prediction is based on automatically extracted ACMs from baseline CT-angiography (CTA). Figure 1 shows an overview of ArterialGNet.

## 2   Methods

*Study Population.* This retrospective study utilized a prospectively maintained database comprising consecutive patients who underwent endovascular thrombectomy at our center between February 2017 and December 2022. We included patients presenting with acute ischemic stroke secondary to a large-vessel occlusion involving either the intracranial segment of the internal carotid artery or the proximal segments of the middle cerebral artery (M1 or M2), provided they had undergone CTA covering the aortic arch to the intracranial vessels. Patients with multiple synchronic occlusions or severe imaging artifacts on CTA that impeded valid analysis were excluded.

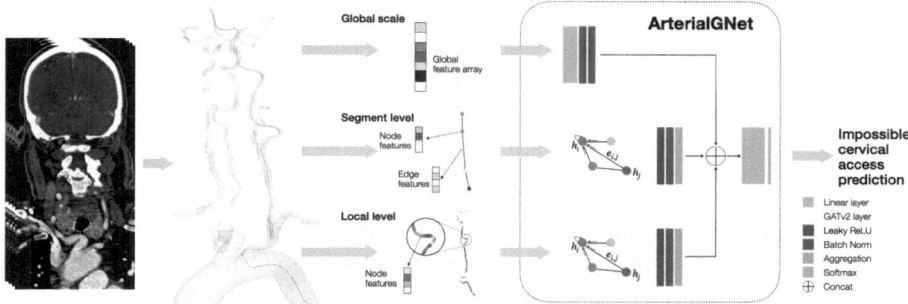

**Fig. 1.** Overview of the supersegment generation from CTA, and schematic view of ArterialGNet with the multi-scale encoder paths.

*Primary Outcome Measure.* The primary outcome measure assessed the inability to access the target intracranial occlusion via the transfemoral access catheter, necessitating the utilization of alternative arterial access for the thrombectomy procedure.

### 2.1   Feature Extraction Preprocessing Pipeline

**Centerline Map and Supersegment Extraction.** Extracranial ACMs were automatically extracted from head-and-neck CTA using a validated vascular analysis framework [16]. This method relies on a trained 3D nnU-Net for artery segmentation [21]. The 3D segmentation object is then used for automatic centerline extraction based on the vascular modelling toolkit (VMTK) [22], and anatomically labelled using a trained graph U-Net [23]. Anatomical labels (e.g., vessel types such as aortic arch, internal carotid artery, etc.) were associated to each individual vascular segment between bifurcations. To ensure that only relevant anatomical information was taken into account, anatomical labels were used to determine vascular pathways from the descending aorta (most proximal point imaged in the CTA) to the internal carotid artery bifurcation. Anatomical label sequences formed by the centerline pathways from the descending aorta to all other endpoints were generated and compared to typical sequences by means of cosine similarity. The sequence with the minimum cosine similarity for the particular occlusion location (anterior circulation, right/left) was selected. The resulting pathway was a centerline without bifurcations, with nodes sampled at a frequency of 0.5 mm$^{-1}$. This was defined as a *supersegment*.

**Multi-scale Featurization.** Supersegments were further processed to generate multi-scale graphs, including a series of geometrical and morphological features. Features were captured at three scales:

- Global scale: a total of 9 features that captured measurements of the whole supersegment were computed. These included the tortuosity index (TI), length, mean vessel diameter and standard deviation (SD), minimum polar component of tangent along the supersegment and overall direction (polar and azimuthal angles for the vector from origin to end of the supersegment). Side of the occlusion and anatomical labels along the supersegment (one-hot encoded) were also included. Features at this scale were encoded as $X_g \in \mathbb{R}^{n_g}$, where $n_g = 9$ is the number of global features.

- Segment scale: an undirected graph $\mathcal{G}_s = (\mathcal{V}_s, \mathcal{E}_s, X_s, H_s)$, where $\mathcal{V}_s = \{v_i\}_{i=1}^{d}$ are the set of nodes, with $d$ as the number of nodes, where $\mathcal{E}_s \in \mathbb{R}^{d \times d}$ is the adjacency matrix, where $X_s \in \mathbb{R}^{d \times n_s}$ are the node features, with $n_s$ as the number of segment node features, and where $H_s \in \mathbb{R}^{f \times g}$ are the edge attributes, with $f$ as the number of edges and $g$ as the number of segment edge attributes, was formed by grouping all consecutive nodes from the supersegment with the same anatomical label (i.e., belonging to the same segment) into one single node. A total of $n_s = 8$ node features were computed (same as global features except for side). Maximum angle differences (cosine, polar and azimuthal) between consecutive segments as well as bifurcation positions were also computed and encoded as edge attributes ($g = 6$).
- Local scale: the supersegment was directly used as an undirected graph $\mathcal{G}_l = (\mathcal{V}_l, \mathcal{E}_l, X_l)$, where $\mathcal{V}_l = \{v_i\}_{i=1}^{h}$ are the nodes, with $h$ as the number of nodes, where $\mathcal{E}_l \in \mathbb{R}^{h \times h}$ is the adjacency matrix, and where $X_l \in \mathbb{R}^{h \times n_l}$ are the node features, with $n_s$ as the number of segment node features, to encode features at a local level. Features were encoded as node attributes. These included the node position, vessel diameter, polar and azimuthal components of tangent vector, curvature, torsion, blanking (a feature derived from VMTK processing that becomes 1 in bifurcations, and is 0 elsewhere), Hounsfield units in the CTA, accumulated length from origin of the supersegment and vessel type (one-hot) for a total of $n_l = 12$ features.

## 2.2 ArterialGNet: Multi-scale Graph Embeddings for Impossible Femoral Access Prediction

Given a supersegment $A_n = \left\{ (X_g, \mathcal{G}_s, \mathcal{G}_l)_n \right\}_{n=1}^{N}$ derived from a vascular CM, where $N$ is the number of examples available we develop a model to predict $y_n$, where $y_n$ is a binary variable defining impossible transfemoral access. In order integrate all the information encoded at different scales, ArterialGNet presents one encoder path for each of the scales. For features encoded at a global level, $X_g$, a multi-layer perceptron (*MLP*)

$$\mathrm{MLP}_K(x) = \mathrm{L}_K(\ldots (\mathrm{L}_2(\mathrm{L}_1(x)))) \tag{1}$$

with $L_K(x) = BatchNorm(LeakyReLU(f_{lin}(x)))$ is a layer of the *MLP*, where $f_{lin}(x)$ is a fully connected layer and $K$ is the number of layers of the *MLP*, was employed to compute feature embeddings $h'_g$:

$$h'_g = \mathrm{MLP}_{N_g}(X_g) \tag{2}$$

The segment-level encoder path was formed by a set of $N_s$ Graph Attention Network (GAT) v2 [24], based on previously introduced GAT layers [25]. Let us assume that every node $i \in \mathcal{V}_s$ with a neighborhood $\mathcal{N}_{s,i} = \{j \in \mathcal{V}_s | i, j \in \mathcal{E}_s\}$ has an initial node representation $h_{s,i}^0 \in \mathbb{R}^{n_s}$, with $h_{s,i}^l \in \mathbb{R}^q$ being the node representation at the $l$-th GATv2 layer, with $l = \{1, 2, \ldots, N_s\}$ and $q$ as the number of hidden dimensions, and every edge $(i, j) \in \mathcal{V}_s$ has an initial edge representation $e_{i,j}^0 \in \mathbb{R}^g$. Then the $h_{s,i}^{l+1} \in \mathbb{R}^q$ node representation is computed as:

$$h_{s,i}^{l+1} = BatchNorm\left( LeakyReLU\left( \alpha_{si,i}^l \Theta_{s,s}^l h_{s,i}^l + \sum_{j \in \mathcal{N}_{s,i}} \alpha_{si,j}^l \Theta_{s,t}^l h_{s,j}^l \right) \right) \tag{3}$$

where $\Theta_{s,s}^l$, $\Theta_{s,t}^l$ are learnable parameters of the $l$-th GATv2 layer, addition represents concatenation and $\alpha_{si,j}^l$ are attention coefficients, defined as:

$$\alpha_{si,j}^l = softmax_j\left(a_s^{lT} LeakyReLU\left(\Theta_{s,s}^l h_{s,i}^l + \Theta_{s,t}^l h_{s,j}^l + \Theta_{s,e}^l e_{i,j}^0\right)\right) \tag{4}$$

where $a_s^l \in \mathbb{R}^{3q}$ and $\Theta_{s,e}^l$ are also learnable parameters. Node representations are aggregated to obtain a final segment-level embedded graph representation $h_s' \in \mathbb{R}^p$:

$$h_s' = \text{AGG}_s\left(h_{s,i}^{N_s}\right) \tag{5}$$

where $\text{AGG}_s(x)$ represents the aggregation function for the segment encoder path.

Similarly, the encoder path for local-level graphs is constructed by successive $N_l$ GATv2 layers. We assume that every node $i \in \mathcal{V}_l$ with a neighborhood $\mathcal{N}_{l,i} = \{j \in \mathcal{V}_l | i, j \in \mathcal{E}_l\}$ has an initial node representation $h_{l,i}^0 \in \mathbb{R}^{n_l}$, with $h_{l,i}^l \in \mathbb{R}^q$ being the node representation at the $l$-th layer with $l = \{1, 2, \ldots, N_l\}$ and $q$ as the number of hidden dimensions. Then the $h_{l,i}^{l+1} \in \mathbb{R}^q$ node representation is computed as in (3), with attention coefficients $\alpha_{li,j}^l$:

$$\alpha_{li,j}^l = softmax_j\left(a_l^{lT} LeakyReLU\left(\Theta_{l,s}^l h_{l,i}^l + \Theta_{l,t}^l h_{l,j}^l\right)\right) \tag{6}$$

where $a_l^l \in \mathbb{R}^{2q}$, $\Theta_{s,s}^l$, $\Theta_{s,t}^l$ are learnable parameters. As for the segment scale, nodes representations are aggregated to yield a final local-level embedded graph representation $h_l' \in \mathbb{R}^p$:

$$h_l' = \text{AGG}_l\left(h_{l,i}^{N_l}\right) \tag{7}$$

where $\text{AGG}_s(x)$ represents the aggregation function for the local encoder path.

Finally, all embedded representations are concatenated and passed to an MLP with the last layer being simply a fully connected layer followed by a softmax layer:

$$p = softmax\left(f_{lin}\left(\text{MLP}_{N_o-1}\left(h_g' + h_s' + h_l'\right)\right)\right) \tag{8}$$

where $N_o$ is the number of layers for the output MLP, and $p \in \mathbb{R}^2$ are the probabilities for the 2 impossible access classes (yes/no). The class $y_{pred}$ was determined based on an optimal threshold computed regarding test results.

**Loss Function.** Learnable parameters are optimized by minimizing the cross-entropy loss, weighted to address class imbalance in our sample:

$$\mathcal{L}_{CE}\left(p, y_{true}\right) = -\sum_{c=1}^C w_c y_c log\left(p_c\right) \tag{9}$$

where $C = 2$ is the number of classes, $w_c = 1/f_c$ are the weights for each class, which are equal to the inverse of the frequency $f_c$ of that class in the dataset and $y_{true} = \{y_c\}_{c=1}^C$ are the one-hot encoded true class labels for each sample.

## 2.3  Experiments

**Model Configuration.** Model hyperparameters were manually tuned. Tuned parameters include the number of layers for each of the scale paths (0, 1, 2), batch size (16, 32, 64, 128), number of hidden channels for the GAT layers (4, 8, 16, 32), aggregation method (min, max, mean, sum), initial learning rate (1e-2, 1e-3, 1e-4), total number of epochs (500, 1000, 2000) and dropout (0.2, 0.5, 0.8, 1.0). Validation performance was used as criterion to select optimal configuration. For simplicity, we only include configurations from the final models. A tendency for quick overfitting was observed which resulted in a final model parameter choice favoring lightweight models. The number of hidden channels was set to $q = 8$, while the aggregation functions $AGG_s = AGG_l$ were set to mean global pooling. The number of layers was set to 1 for all encoder paths ($N_g = N_s = N_l = 1$) and output layer ($N_o = 1$). Versions of ArterialGNet with no global-level encoder ($N_g = 0$, ArterialGNet[sl]), no segment-level encoder ($N_s = 0$, ArterialGNet[gl]), no local-level encoder ($N_l = 0$, ArterialGNet[gs]), and only local-level encoder ($N_g = 0$, $N_s = 0$, ArterialGNet[l]) were also tested.

**Training Setup.** Models were trained for a total of 500 epochs. A batch size of 64 was used. ADAM optimizer [26] was used ($\beta_0 = 0.9$, $\beta_1 = 0.999$), with an initial learning rate of 1e-3, and a weight decay of 1e-3. A polynomial learning rate decay with an exponent of 0.9 was used. A dropout of 0.8 was used during training. Accuracy was used to monitor training and validation performance during training.

**Validation Setup.** For testing, 20% of the dataset was held out, and the rest of the data was used for 5-fold cross-validation. In order to mitigate the high variability of the classification metrics due to a small number of positive test examples, this was repeated 5 times, varying the testing set as in 5-fold cross validation for testing. This yielded a total of 25 models (5 for each validation fold, for each of the 5 testing sets). Final included metrics result from a model ensembling of the 5 validation folds, averaging final predictions for each testing sample. A batch size of 1 was used during testing.

**Software.** Experiments were performed on an Nvidia A5000 GPU. ArterialGNet was implemented in PyTorch Geometric [27], PyTorch and sklearn, on Python 3.12.

**Evaluation.** Area under the receiver operating characteristic (*AUROC*) was used as the primary indicator of model performance. Sensitivity (*Sens*), specificity (*Spec*), $F_1$ score (*$F_1$*) and Matthew's correlation coefficient (*MCC*) were used as indicators of classification performance. Youden's index maximization was used as criteria for optimal threshold selection for all testing sets independently. The model was compared to a previous internal model trained on the same dataset based on a random forest binary classifier with extreme gradient boosting (XGBRF) [28] that was optimized for this task. The baseline model was evaluated using the same 5-by-5 cross-validation setup. DeLong test was implemented to evaluate differences between receiver operating characteristic (ROC) curves.

# 3   Results

A total of 493 patients were included, including 19 (3.9%) patients that presented impossible transfemoral access. Classification metrics for all tested models and other relevant literature are reported in Table 1. A comparison between ROC and precision-recall (PR) curves of the XGBRF and the ArterialGNet models is observed in Fig. 2.

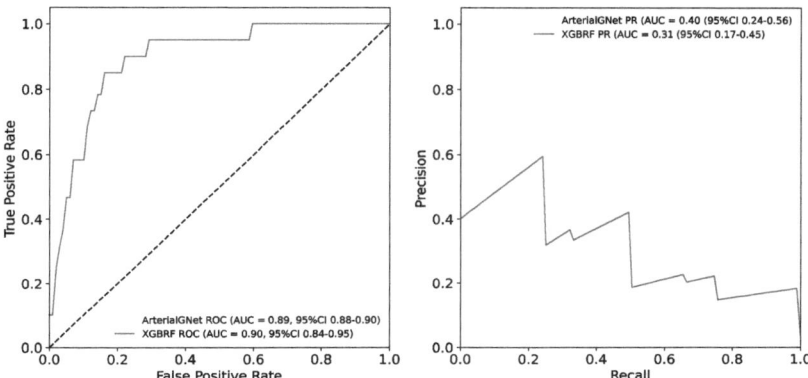

**Fig. 2.** ROC (left) and precision-recall (PR, right) curves for the ArterialGNet (blue) and the XGBRF (red) models for impossible access prediction. Semi-transparent bands show 95%CI. (Color figure online)

**Table 1.** Comparison of classification metrics across different ArterialGNet configurations, and the also compared to an XGBRF baseline optimized for this task as well as previous literature. Mean results averaged across testing sets as well as 95%CI are reported for all metrics. gs: global + segment. gl: global + local. l: local. sl: segment + local.

| Model | N (%imp) | AUROC | Sens | Spec | $F_1$ | MCC |
|---|---|---|---|---|---|---|
| Holswilder 2023 [14] | 1998 (7.0%) | 0.69 (0.62–0.75) | — | — | — | — |
| XGBRF [28] | 493 (3.9%) | **0.90 (0.84–0.95)** | **0.95 (0.86–1.00)** | 0.82 (0.77–0.88) | 0.32 (0.24–0.40) | 0.38 (0.30–0.47) |
| **ArterialGNet[gs]** | 493 (3.9%) | 0.71 (0.60–0.83) | 0.80 (0.64–0.96) | 0.75 (0.64–0.87) | 0.22 (0.17–0.28) | 0.26 (0.21–0.31) |
| **ArterialGNet[gl]** | 493 (3.9%) | 0.89 (0.88–0.91) | 0.90 (0.79–1.00) | 0.82 (0.72–0.93) | 0.38 (0.20–0.56) | 0.43 (0.28–0.58) |
| **ArterialGNet[l]** | 493 (3.9%) | 0.89 (0.87–0.91) | 0.90 (0.79–1.00) | 0.82 (0.71–0.93) | 0.39 (0.19–0.60) | 0.43 (0.28–0.57) |
| **ArterialGNet[sl]** | 493 (3.9%) | **0.90 (0.89–0.90)** | 0.90 (0.79–1.00) | 0.83 (0.73–0.94) | 0.41 (0.21–0.60) | 0.45 (0.29–0.61) |
| **ArterialGNet** | 493 (3.9%) | 0.89 (0.88–0.90) | 0.90 (0.79–1.00) | **0.85 (0.74–0.96)** | **0.43 (0.24–0.62)** | **0.47 (0.31–0.63)** |

Results show how both ArterialGNet and the XGBRF baseline model dramatically improve discrimination ability over previously reported logistic regression models based on manual feature computation [14] (up to + 0.21 on *AUROC*). Compared to the XGBRF baseline, ArterialGNet presents higher $F_1$ and *MCC* as well as similar *AUROC* with reduced variability. Difference between ROC curves evaluated over the whole set (out-of-fold samples) were non-significant (DeLong test p = 0.963). When comparing Arterial-GNet configurations, we can see how local-level features were the most influential on the final model performance (Table 1). ArterialGNet[gs] shows poor discrimination ability compared to all other configurations that include a local-level encoder path. Differences across configurations that incorporated the local-level encoder were minimal.

The processing pipeline necessary to generate the centerline graphs took a median time of 178.2s (IQR 150.7–209.8 s) per case, including segmentation, centerline extraction, vessel labelling and feature extraction. Processing time with ArterialGNet is minimal (~0.01s per case). Overall, processing times would fit in the context of acute ischemic stroke, making it compatible with prospective implementation.

## 4 Discussion

We present ArterialGNet, a GNN based on GATv2 able to input feature embeddings of arterial centerline segments at multiple-scales, that achieves state-of-the-art performance on impossible femoral access prediction in the context of mechanical thrombectomy for stroke treatment.

Predicting impossible catheterization of the cervical arteries prior to arterial access can enable a quantitative and patient-specific approach for access selection before arterial puncture. This may help reduce intervention times in selected cohorts, leading to enhanced treatment effect and improved clinical outcomes.

Compared to previous models employed for impossible access prediction, GNNs such as ArterialGNet present some key properties that elevate them for this specific context. ACMs are normally used for automatic computation processes to extract higher level features that are later fed to classical machine learning and probability models. The quality of this feature computation step is key to the final model's performance and robustness, which is not always an easy task. Moreover, this reliance on handcrafted features restricts the flexibility of the models, making them less adaptable to other similar tasks such as impossible transradial access prediction. Even in absence of a significant leap in performance of the model, these qualities make ArterialGNet an interesting proposition. Given the simplicity of the graph structure (a 1-dimensional graph), there may be simpler models that may also be capable of delivering similar performance for impossible access prediction such as recurrent neural networks or other types of networks designed for series processing. However, this has not been explored in this work.

Main limitations of this work are the absence of an external test set or the high class imbalance (which reflects clinical reality), which may hinder generalizability of results. The lack of inclusion of relevant factors such as operator experience or device setup used is also a limitation, as these factors may influence access.

The inclusion of larger-scale features resulted in a marginal, non-significant improvement of the predictive ability of the model (all DeLong test $p > 0.05$ between ArterialGNet and all other variants). Future work will focus on redesigning architectural elements to leverage global and segment-scale features, adding intermediate-level scales (i.e., centerline graphs sampled at reduced density to integrate intermediate-level features), further validating the model with external data from other centers and integrating ACMs from radial access for further assessment. Inclusion of posterior circulation pathways and exploring the use of attention maps as potential methods for explainability are other foci of future work.

# 5   Conclusion

This study presents ArterialGNet, a novel model for impossible transfemoral access prediction based on CTA in the context of mechanical thrombectomy for stroke treatment. The model is able to achieve high discrimination ability ($AUROC = 0.89$, 95%CI 0.88–0.90), with high sensitivity (0.90, 95%CI 0.79–1.00) and specificity (0.85, 95%CI 0.74–0.96). ArterialGNet achieved similar results to a previous baseline model, with key design advantages. Effective and fast predictions could aid in decision making towards arterial access choice endovascular interventions procedures, ultimately reducing procedural times and improving clinical outcomes on a patient-specific basis.

**Acknowledgements.** This work was partially supported by the Catalan Health Department (Departament de Salut, Generalitat de Catalunya, PERIS PIF-Salut 2021, grant number SLT017/20/000180) and the Spanish Health Institute Carlos III (Instituto de Salud Carlos III, Ministerio de Ciencia e Innovación, Gobierno de España) with a PI21 grant (PI21/01967).

# References

1. Fischer, U., et al.: Thrombectomy alone versus intravenous alteplase plus thrombectomy in patients with stroke: an open-label, blinded-outcome, randomised non-inferiority trial. Lancet **400**, 104–115 (2022)
2. Kaesmacher, J., et al.: Reasons for reperfusion failures in stent-retriever-based thrombectomy: registry analysis and proposal of a classification system. Am. J. Neuroradiol. **39**, 1848–1853 (2018)
3. Leischner, H., et al.: Reasons for failed endovascular recanalization attempts in stroke patients. J. Neurointerv. Surg. **11**, 439–442 (2019)
4. Penide, J., et al.: Systematic review on endovascular access to intracranial arteries for mechanical thrombectomy in acute ischemic stroke. Clin. Neuroradiol. (2021). https://doi.org/10.1007/s00062-021-01100-7
5. Kaymaz, Z.O., Nikoubashman, O., Brockmann, M.A., Wiesmann, M., Brockmann, C.: Influence of carotid tortuosity on internal carotid artery access time in the treatment of acute ischemic stroke. Interv. Neuroradiol. **23**, 583–588 (2017)
6. Dumont, T.M., Bina, R.W.: Difficult vascular access anatomy associated with decreased success of revascularization in emergent thrombectomy. J. Vasc. Interv. Neurol. **10**, 11–14 (2018)
7. Mokin, M., et al.: Semi-automated measurement of vascular tortuosity and its implications for mechanical thrombectomy performance. Neuroradiology (2020). https://doi.org/10.1007/s00234-020-02525-6
8. Benson, J.C., Brinjikji, W., Messina, S.A., Lanzino, G., Kallmes, D.F.: Cervical internal carotid artery tortuosity: a morphologic analysis of patients with acute ischemic stroke. Interv. Neuroradiol. **26**, 216–221 (2020)
9. Rosa, J.A., et al.: Aortic and supra-aortic arterial tortuosity and access technique: Impact on time to device deployment in stroke thrombectomy. Interv. Neuroradiol. **27**, 419–426 (2021)
10. Gomez-Paz, S., et al.: Tortuosity index predicts early successful reperfusion and affects functional status after thrombectomy for stroke. World Neurosurg. **152**, e1–e10 (2021)
11. Holswilder, G., et al.: The prognostic value of extracranial vascular characteristics on procedural duration and revascularization success in endovascularly treated acute ischemic stroke patients. Eur. Stroke J. **7**, 48–56 (2022)

12. Elfil, M., et al.: Transradial versus transfemoral access for mechanical thrombectomy: a systematic review and meta-analysis. Stroke Vasc. Interv. Neurol. **3**, 1–14 (2023)
13. Hernandez, D., et al.: Radial versus femoral access for mechanical thrombectomy in stroke patients: a non-inferiority randomized clinical trial. Stroke **55**(Suppl\_1), A81−A81 (2024)
14. Holswilder, G., et al.: Development and validation of a prediction model for failure of the transfemoral approach of endovascular treatment for large vessel occlusion acute ischemic stroke. Cerebrovasc. Dis. (2023). https://doi.org/10.1159/000535758
15. Snelling, B.M., et al.: Unfavorable vascular anatomy is associated with increased revascularization time and worse outcome in anterior circulation thrombectomy. World Neurosurg. **120**, e976–e983 (2018)
16. Canals, P., et al.: A fully automatic method for vascular tortuosity feature extraction in the supra-aortic region: unraveling possibilities in stroke treatment planning. Comput. Med. Imaging Graph. **104**, 102170 (2023)
17. Chen, L., Hatsukami, T., Hwang, J.N., Yuan, C.: Automated intracranial artery labeling using a graph neural network and hierarchical refinement. arXiv 1, 1–11 (2020)
18. Yao, L., et al.: Graph convolutional network based point cloud for head and neck vessel labeling. Lect. Notes Comput. Sci. (including Subser. Lect. Notes Artif. Intell. Lect. Notes Bioinformatics) 12436 LNCS, pp. 474–483 (2020)
19. Yao, L., et al.: TaG-Net: Topology-Aware Graph Network for Vessel Labeling. in Imaging Systems for GI Endoscopy, and Graphs in Biomedical Image Analysis: First MICCAI Workshop, ISGIE 2022, and Fourth MICCAI Workshop, GRAIL 2022, Held in Conjunction with MICCAI 2022, Singapore, September 18, 2022, Proceedings pp. 108–117 (Springer-Verlag, Berlin, Heidelberg, 2022). https://doi.org/10.1007/978-3-031-21083-9_11
20. Hong, S.W., et al.: Automated in-depth cerebral arterial labelling using cerebrovascular vasculature reframing and deep neural networks. Sci. Rep. **13**, 1–14 (2023)
21. Isensee, F., Jaeger, P.F., Kohl, S.A.A., Petersen, J., Maier-Hein, K.H.: NnU-Net: a self-configuring method for deep learning-based biomedical image segmentation. Nat. Methods **18**, 203–211 (2021)
22. Antiga, L., Ene-Iordache, B., Remuzzi, A.: Centerline computation and geometric analysis of branching tubular surfaces with application to blood vessel modeling. Wscg (2003)
23. Gao, H., Ji, S.: Graph U-nets. In: 36th International Conference Machine Learning ICML 2019 2019-June, pp. 3651–3660 (2019)
24. Brody, S., Alon, U., Yahav, E.: How Attentive are Graph Attention Networks? ICLR 2022 abs/2105.1, (2021)
25. Veličković, P., et al.: Graph attention networks. In: 6th International Conference Learning Represent. ICLR 2018 - Conf. Track Proc. pp. 1–12 (2018)
26. Kingma, D.P., Ba, J.L.: Adam: A method for stochastic optimization. In: 3rd International Conference Learning Represent. ICLR 2015 - Conf. Track Proc. pp. 1–15 (2015)
27. Fey, M., Lenssen, J.E.: Fast Graph Representation Learning with PyTorch Geometric. at https://github.com/pyg-team/pytorch_geometric (2019)
28. Canals, P., et al.: Deep learning-based model for difficult transfemoral access prediction compared with human assessment in stroke thrombectomy. J. Neurointerv. Surg. 1–7 (2024) https://doi.org/10.1136/jnis-2024-021718

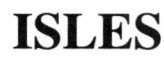

**ISLES**

# Spatio-Temporal Deep Learning for Final Infarct Prediction Using Acute Stroke CT Perfusion Data

Kimberly Amador[1,2,3]($\boxtimes$), Anthony J. Winder[2], and Nils D. Forkert[2,3,4]

[1] Biomedical Engineering Graduate Program, University of Calgary, Calgary, Canada
[2] Department of Radiology, University of Calgary, Calgary, Canada
[3] Hotchkiss Brain Institute, University of Calgary, Calgary, Canada
`kimberlyalejandra.am@ucalgary.ca`
[4] Alberta Children's Hospital Research Institute, University of Calgary, Calgary, Canada

**Abstract.** Accurate prediction of the tissue outcome is crucial for guiding treatment decisions in acute ischemic stroke (AIS). Spatio-temporal (4D) Computed Tomography Perfusion (CTP) provides detailed insights into cerebral blood flow dynamics, which are essential for predicting final infarct regions. However, its high-dimensional and noisy nature presents challenges for direct prediction. In this study, we evaluate a deep learning model that fully leverages 4D CTP data for predicting tissue outcomes. The model integrates a shared-weight convolutional neural network (CNN) encoder, a Transformer encoder, and a CNN decoder to capture both spatial and temporal dependencies within the data. We evaluated this approach on a multicenter dataset of 143 patients from the ISLES 2024 challenge. The results reveal a Dice score of 0.20, an absolute volume difference of 17 ml, a mean lesion count difference of 19, and a lesion-wise F1-Score of 0.02, underscoring both the potential and challenges of directly utilizing 4D CTP data for final infarct prediction.

**Keywords:** Stroke · Final Infarct Prediction · CTP · Deep Learning

## 1 Introduction

Acute ischemic stroke (AIS) is caused by an arterial occlusion that restricts blood flow to the brain, leading to rapid neurological deterioration and even death [3]. Accurately estimating the extent of irreversibly damaged (infarct core) and potentially salvageable (penumbra) brain tissue is critical for guiding treatment decisions in AIS [8]. Spatio-temporal (4D) Computed Tomography Perfusion (CTP) is an imaging technique that measures cerebral blood flow dynamics by capturing a series of 3D CT images over time following the injection of a contrast agent [6]. In clinical practice, 4D CTP scans are typically postprocessed using

---

K. Amador, A.J. Winder — Shared first authorship

R. Su et al. (Eds.): ISLES 2024/SWITCH 2024, LNCS 15408, pp. 83–88, 2025.
https://doi.org/10.1007/978-3-031-81101-2_9

deconvolution algorithms to generate 3D perfusion parameter maps for clinical decision-making, such as cerebral blood flow (CBF) and time-to-maximum (Tmax). While computationally efficient, this approach oversimplifies the complex pathophysiology of AIS [4]. In recent years, machine learning has emerged as a promising option to guide AIS treatment decisions [7]. While early deep learning models focused on tissue outcome prediction using perfusion maps, recent research has demonstrated that directly using 4D CTP data for this purpose leads to superior results [1,2,10,14,15]. Within this context, advanced techniques such as channel-wise convolutions [10], temporal convolutional networks (TCNs) [1,15], and attention-based methods [2,14] have been proposed to leverage the full spatio-temporal information contained in 4D CTP data. Among these, attention-based methods are particularly notable due to their ability to dynamically prioritize and weigh the relevance of different time points and regions, enabling them to effectively capture long-range dependencies and subtle temporal patterns in the data.

The Ischemic Stroke Lesion Segmentation (ISLES) 2024 challenge [9,11] offers an opportunity to benchmark methods for tissue outcome prediction using acute stroke CT imaging modalities (*e.g.,* CT angiography, non-contrast CT, 4D CTP) and clinical data. In this work, we evaluate the effectiveness and generalizability of our previously proposed model [2] using data from the ISLES 2024 challenge.

## 2   Methods

The goal for this challenge is to predict a binary mask of the final infarct using acute 4D CTP imaging data. Building upon our previous work [2], we applied and tested a model architecture consisting of three modules, as shown in Fig. 1: (i) a *convolutional neural network (CNN) encoder* with shared weights across time to extract high-level spatial features from each time point, (ii) a *Transformer encoder* to capture the temporal dependencies, and (iii) a *CNN decoder* to upsample the encoded features and predict the probability of each voxel developing infarction. For this study, only minor adjustments to the original model were made to improve the model's computational efficiency by reducing the number of blocks in the encoder-decoder from five to four. Moreover, we adapted the original model to the ISLES 2024 challenge dataset by reparameterizing the input layer to accept image slices with larger size (416×416 voxels). To further optimize efficiency and accommodate varying slice numbers across patients, the model processes slices independently over time, reducing the 3D+time problem to multiple 2D+time problems. Code is available on GitHub.

### 2.1   Model Architecture

**CNN Encoder.** The input 4D CTP sequence is processed by a CNN encoder with shared weights applied uniformly across all time points. This weight-sharing approach enhances parameter efficiency and reduces computational costs. Each

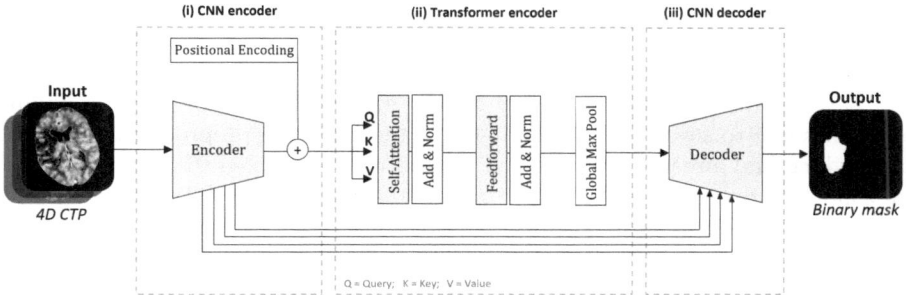

**Fig. 1.** Overview of the proposed model for tissue outcome prediction.

encoder is composed of four blocks, each containing two convolutional layers with ReLU activations followed by a downsampling layer. The resulting low-dimensional representations from each time point are flattened and then concatenated along the temporal dimension, with positional encoding [13] added to provide information regarding the order of time points.

**Transformer Encoder.** The extracted embedding matrix is processed by a vanilla Transformer encoder [13] to capture temporal dependencies among time points. Starting with a multi-head self-attention layer, the Transformer evaluates the importance of each time point relative to others using scaled dot-product attention. This is followed by a feed-forward network with two dense layers and a GELU activation in between. Layer normalization and residual connections are incorporated to stabilize training and ensure efficient gradient flow. As a result, the Transformer encoder outputs a set of contextualized embeddings for each time point, reflecting learned relationships and interactions. A global max-pooling layer reduces these embeddings to a single feature representation, which is reshaped into a 2D image for the CNN decoder.

**CNN Decoder.** The reshaped 2D image is fed into the CNN decoder, which progressively upsamples the feature representations to restore the original spatial resolution for pixel-level predictions. The decoder mirrors the structure of the encoder blocks, except for the last one, which comprises two convolutional layers and a softmax layer. During upsampling, skip connections between the encoder and decoder provide localized spatial information. This is achieved by concatenating the absolute differences between skip connections, as proposed in [1], further emphasizing variations between time points while reducing computational costs. Finally, the probability maps resulting from the softmax layer are thresholded at 0.5, to produce the binary final infarct mask.

## 2.2  Dataset

The proposed method was evaluated on a multicenter database consisting of 150 AIS patients made available for the ISLES 2024 challenge [9]. After excluding 7 patients due to severe motion artifacts, we utilized the preprocessed 4D CTP data, which had already been defaced, temporally resampled to 1 frame per second, motion-corrected, and linearly co-registered to the NCCT. We performed additional preprocessing to ensure that all images share a common voxel spacing and image extents. First, we linearly resampled the images to a uniform voxel spacing of [0.45, 0.45, 2.0] and image extents of [416, 416] in the axial plane. Voxels with intensity >100 HU were masked out to remove the skull. Next, the contrast signal was isolated by averaging the first three time points and subtracting this average from the entire sequence. We standardized the sequence length by extracting a 32-second window from each scan, centering the temporal window around the time point with the greatest mean enhancement. Finally, Z-score normalization was applied across all voxels and time points to ensure uniform contrast dynamics, making the contrast agent dynamics more comparable between patients.

## 2.3  Experimental Setup

The model was trained end-to-end using a Dice loss function [12] to maximize the overlap between the predicted and ground truth segmentations. The dataset was divided into 80% training and 20% testing samples, with stratified sampling at the patient level to ensure a balanced representation of final infarct volumes in both sets. The parameters of the final training setup were empirically defined as follows: 100 epochs, batch size of 4, initial learning rate of 0.001, and Adam optimizer with a step-based learning rate decay (reduced by a factor of 0.25 every 15 epochs). Model weights were initialized from a pre-training session that used the same parameters described above in conjunction with a private dataset. The Transformer encoder was configured with one layer and eight attention heads. To prevent over-fitting and enhance model generalization, an L2 regularization was applied to each layer. The model was implemented in Python using TensorFlow and trained on an NVIDIA GeForce RTX 3090 with 24 GB memory.

## 3  Results

We evaluated the model using Dice score, absolute volume difference, absolute lesion count difference, and lesion-wise F1-Score. These metrics were calculated using *panoptica* [5], a tool for 2D and 3D segmentation evaluation. Metrics were first computed per patient and then averaged across the entire testing set. The final results, presented as mean (standard deviation), are as follows: Dice score of 0.20 (0.23), absolute volume difference of 17 (25) ml, lesion count difference of 19 (33), and lesion-wise F1-Score of 0.02 (0.07).

# 4 Discussion

In this work, we evaluated the performance of our proposed spatio-temporal deep learning model for final infarct prediction using 4D CTP data from the ISLES 2024 challenge. The results underscore both the potential and challenges associated with directly leveraging 4D CTP data for this task. Particularly, the relatively low Dice score and lesion-wise F1-score indicate that, while the model captures some aspects of the underlying pathology, there remains room for improvement in accurately predicting the exact spatial extent of the infarct. Despite these challenges, a key advantage of using 4D CTP data directly lies in its ability to preserve the temporal dimension, enabling the model to monitor blood flow changes over time. This dynamic approach provides a richer feature set, capturing subtle perfusion variations that static imaging methods, such as perfusion maps, might overlook. Direct CTP analysis may, for example, benefit multi-modality models. Moreover, this spatio-temporal approach streamlines the clinical workflow and reduces the likelihood of human error, potentially making the analysis faster and more efficient.

Several limitations must be acknowledged. First, the restricted field of view (*i.e.*, limited number of slices) in 4D CTP imaging may prevent the model from capturing the full extent of ischemic damage, potentially impacting the lesion overlap accuracy. This problem could be mitigated by incorporating additional imaging modalities, such as CT angiography and non-contrast CT, which provide a full coverage of the brain's vascular and structural tissues. Second, the proposed method relies solely on imaging data. Thus, integrating clinical information (*e.g.*, demographics, risk factors, neurological assessments) could enhance the model's robustness and precision, enabling a more comprehensive evaluation of the data.

**Acknowledgments.** This work is supported by the Canada Research Chairs Program, the River Fund at Calgary Foundation, and the Heart and Stroke Foundation (G-24-0037894).

**Disclosure of Interests.** The authors have no competing interests to declare that are relevant to the content of this article.

# References

1. Amador, K., Wilms, M., Winder, A., Fiehler, J., Forkert, N.D.: Predicting treatment-specific lesion outcomes in acute ischemic stroke from 4D CT perfusion imaging using spatio-temporal convolutional neural networks. Med. Image Anal. **82**, 102610 (2022). https://doi.org/10.1016/j.media.2022.102610
2. Amador, K., Winder, A., Fiehler, J., Wilms, M., Forkert, N.D.: Hybrid spatio-temporal transformer network for predicting ischemic stroke lesion outcomes from 4d ct perfusion imaging. In: Medical Image Computing and Computer-Assisted Intervention – MICCAI 2022, pp. 644–654. Springer Nature Switzerland (2022). https://doi.org/10.1007/978-3-031-16437-8_62
3. Chan, B.P., Albers, G.W.: Acute ischemic stroke. Curr. Treat. Options Neurol.**1**(2), 83–95 (1999). https://doi.org/10.1007/s11940-999-0009-5

4. Flottmann, F., et al.: Ct-perfusion stroke imaging: a threshold-free probabilistic approach to predict infarct volume compared to traditional ischemic thresholds. Sci. Rep. **7**(1), 1–10 (2017). https://doi.org/10.1038/s41598-017-06882-w
5. Kofler, F., et al.: Panoptica – instance-wise evaluation of 3d semantic and instance segmentation maps (2023). arXiv:2312.02608, https://arxiv.org/abs/2312.02608
6. Konstas, A.A., Wintermark, M., Lev, M.H.: Ct perfusion imaging in acute stroke. Neuroimaging Clin. N. Am. **21**(2), 215–238 (2011). https://doi.org/10.1016/j.nic.2011.01.008
7. Lo Vercio, L., Amador, K., Bannister, J.J., Crites, S., Gutierrez, A., MacDonald, M.E., et al.: Supervised machine learning tools: a tutorial for clinicians. J. Neural Eng. **17**(6), 062001 (2020). https://doi.org/10.1088/1741-2552/abbff2
8. Neumann-Haefelin, T., Wittsack, H.J., Wenserski, F., Siebler, M., Seitz, R.J., Mödder, U., et al.: Diffusion- and perfusion-weighted MRI. Stroke **30**(8), 1591–1597 (1999). https://doi.org/10.1161/01.str.30.8.1591
9. Riedel, E.O., et al.: Isles 2024: the first longitudinal multimodal multi-center real-world dataset in (sub-)acute stroke (2024). arXiv:2408.11142, https://arxiv.org/abs/2408.11142
10. Robben, D., et al.: Prediction of final infarct volume from native ct perfusion and treatment parameters using deep learning. Med. Image Anal. **59**, 101589 (2020). https://doi.org/10.1016/j.media.2019.101589
11. de la Rosa, E., et al.: Isles'24: improving final infarct prediction in ischemic stroke using multimodal imaging and clinical data (2024). arXiv:2408.10966, https://arxiv.org/abs/2408.10966
12. Sudre, C.H., Li, W., Vercauteren, T., Ourselin, S., Jorge Cardoso, M.: Generalised dice overlap as a deep learning loss function for highly unbalanced segmentations. In: Deep Learning in Medical Image Analysis and Multimodal Learning for Clinical Decision Support – DLMIA ML-CDS 2017, pp. 240–248. Springer International Publishing (2017). https://doi.org/10.1007/978-3-319-67558-9_28
13. Vaswani, A., et al.: Attention is all you need. In: Neural Information Processing Systems – NeurIPS 2017, pp. 5998–6008 (2017)
14. de Vries, L., Emmer, B.J., Majoie, C.B., Marquering, H.A., Gavves, E.: Perfu-net: baseline infarct estimation from ct perfusion source data for acute ischemic stroke. Med. Image Anal. **85**, 102749 (2023). https://doi.org/10.1016/j.media.2023.102749
15. Winder, A.J., Wilms, M., Amador, K., Flottmann, F., Fiehler, J., Forkert, N.D.: Predicting the tissue outcome of acute ischemic stroke from acute 4D computed tomography perfusion imaging using temporal features and deep learning. Front. Neurosci. **16**, 1009654 (2022). https://doi.org/10.3389/fnins.2022.1009654

# Utilizing Baseline Infarct and Penumbra Masks to Improve NCCT and CTA Based Final Infarct Prediction

Mahsa Mojtahedi(✉)(iD), Laura van Poppel(iD), Lucas de Vries(iD), Bart Emmer(iD), Charles Majoie(iD), and Henk Marquering(iD)

Amsterdam UMC, location AMC, Amsterdam, AZ 1105, The Netherlands
{s.m.mojtahedi,l.m.vanpoppel,lucas.devries,b.j.emmer,
c.b.majoie,h.a.marquering}@amsterdamumc.nl

**Abstract.** Estimating the final ischemic lesions is important for guiding treatment decisions in stroke patients. The baseline infarct and penumbra are two of the most important pre-interventional biomarkers for prognosticating stroke patients. Baseline CT scans implicitly contain information about these biomarkers. This study evaluates the added value of including NCCT/CTA-based baseline lesion masks as input to predict the final infarct. Given that CTP scans are less accessible than other CT modalities, particularly in medically underserved areas, we analyze two scenarios: when baseline CTP scans are available and when they are not. Using the nnU-Net framework, we observe a 16% improvement in Dice when baseline lesion masks are added in the absence of CTP. However, when CTP maps are included, the addition of baseline lesion masks is no longer beneficial.

**Keywords:** Ischemic stroke · Final infarct · Medical image segmentation · CT scans

## 1 Introduction

In stroke management, understanding the progression of the ischemic lesion can provide valuable prognostic information and aid clinicians in determining the most appropriate treatment strategy. The final infarct prediction is influenced by multiple factors, including baseline biomarkers, such as age and lesion characteristics; treatment selection and outcomes, and post-interventional variables, such as hemorrhagic transformations [1].

Given that the baseline condition of a patient strongly influences infarction progression, pre-interventional information can potentially be used to estimate the final infarct. One of the main sources of information on the patient's baseline condition is radiological brain imaging. Non-Contrast Computed Tomography (NCCT) and Computed Tomography Angiography (CTA) scans provide

---

L. van Poppel, L. de Vries—These authors contributed equally to this work.

R. Su et al. (Eds.): ISLES 2024/SWITCH 2024, LNCS 15408, pp. 89–94, 2025.
https://doi.org/10.1007/978-3-031-81101-2_10

information on early ischemic tissue changes, the presence of hemorrhage, and collateral capacity. Additionally, Computed Tomography Perfusion (CTP) scans contain information about cerebral perfusion and can be used to assess baseline lesions and tissue at risk [2]. However, a main disadvantage of CTP is that it is not as widely available as NCCT and CTA, especially in medically underserved areas. Furthermore, CTP scans are more prone to artefacts than other CT modalities [3], and not all CTP scanners offer full brain coverage.

The volume and location of baseline infarct and penumbra are key imaging biomarkers for stroke prognosis [4]. Since NCCT and CTA contain information on the baseline ischemic lesion [5], a model that uses these scans as input *implicitly* has access to information on the infarct and penumbra. However, such a model still needs to learn to utilize this implicit information effectively. In this study, we explore whether *explicitly* incorporating baseline infarct and penumbra segmentations derived from NCCT and CTA scans as additional input enhances the accuracy of predicting the final infarct. We consider two scenarios: when baseline CTP scans are available and when they are not. If CTP is available, we explore the value of adding an NCCT/CTA-based lesion mask alongside CTP maps as input in predicting the final infarct.

## 2   Methods

We evaluate the added value of providing a final infarct segmentation model with an NCCT/CTA-based baseline lesion mask as input.

*Part 1—NCCT/CTA models:* We evaluate the scenario in which CTP is unavailable. We compare the performance of a final infarct prediction model utilizing only NCCT and CTA scans (experiment **A**) with the performance of a model utilizing NCCT, CTA and NCCT/CTA based baseline infarct and penumbra masks (experiment **B**).

*Part 2—including CTP:* In the second part, we include the CTP perfusion maps as well. We compare the performance of a model trained on NCCT, CTA and all the CTP perfusion maps (experiment **C**) with a model trained on NCCT, CTA and CTP perfusion maps plus the baseline lesion masks obtained from NCCT and CTA (experiment **D**). Here we hypothesize that the static higher-quality NCCT and CTA images have added value in characterizing the baseline infarct to the dynamic, but lower-quality CTP images.

### 2.1   Model

U-Net is a widely used segmentation architecture. The nnU-Net framework was developed to standardize data processing, hyperparameter tuning, and training of a U-Net, and it has outperformed hand-crafted solutions in several medical image segmentation challenges [6]. We selected nnU-Net for our experiments due to its optimal performance without a need for manual hyperparameter tuning and its high reproducibility; allowing us to focus on the impact of input type on final infarct segmentation accuracy. We use the 3D full resolution setting in nnU-Net version 2. All nnU-Nets were trained for 500 epochs.

## 2.2  Data

We use the ISLES 2024 dataset [7,8]. This dataset includes final infarct segmentation masks annotated on diffusion weighted imaging (DWI). We use the first (46 cases) and second (47 cases) batches of the ISLES 2024 dataset for training and 5-fold cross-validation; and the third batch (57 cases) for testing.

*Baseline lesion masks:* In this study, we use a previously developed in-house model to produce the baseline lesion masks. This model is an nnU-Net that takes NCCT and CTA as input and produces a mask containing labels for baseline infarct core and penumbra. It was trained with CTP masks as ground truth.

*CTP perfusion maps:* We use all the perfusion maps provided in the ISLES 2024 dataset for the CTP-including models. The perfusion maps include relative cerebral blood flow (rCBF), relative cerebral blood volume (rCBV), mean transit time (MTT), and time to maximum (TMAX).

*Preprocessing:* We use the co-registered scans provided by ISLES 2024. For all scans and CTP maps, we set the background values to zero. Additionally, we clip the voxel values between the following intervals: NCCT [0, 100] HU, CTA [0, 200] HU, rCBF [0, 400] %, rCBV [0, 400] %, MTT [0, 20] s, TMAX [0, 20] s. During nnU-Net preprocessing, we apply global normalization for NCCT and CTA, and per-channel z-scoring for the CTP maps.

# 3  Results

*Part 1—NCCT/CTA models:* Both experiments in this part use NCCT and CTA as input, with experiment **B** also including baseline lesion masks. Results are shown in Table 1. Both models underestimate the infarct, and the segmentations have a low overlap with the the DWI-based ground truth. However, adding baseline lesion masks improves the average Dice score by 16% ($\frac{(Dice_B - Dice_A) \times 100}{Dice_A}$). While both models miss many connected components present in the ground truth, the inclusion of baseline masks improves the detection rate of these components. Although the volumetric difference has lower error in experiment **B**, the absolute volumetric differences between the two experiments are similar.

**Table 1.** Final infarct segmentation results for models *excluding* CTP. All values are averaged over the test set. 95% confidence intervals are reported. A positive volumetric difference indicates an overestimation of infarct volume compared to the DWI-based ground truth. BL mask: baseline lesion mask, Exp.: experiment name. % detected CC: percentage of connected components in the ground truth that overlaps with the prediction.

| Exp. | Input list | Dice score ↑ | Surface Dice ↑ | Volumetric difference (ml) | Absolute volumetric difference (ml)↓ | % detected CC ↑ |
|---|---|---|---|---|---|---|
| **A** | NCCT+CTA | $17.7 \pm 6.5$ | $19.8 \pm 7.2$ | -21.0 ± 8.3 | $21.4 \pm 8.2$ | $11.8\% \pm 4.9$ |
| **B** | NCCT+CTA+BL mask | **$20.5 \pm 6.6$** | **$22.4 \pm 7.1$** | **$-15.7 \pm 9$** | **$20.5 \pm 8.4$** | **$15.1\% \pm 5.8$** |

*Part 2—including CTP:* Table 2 shows the results of the models that included CTP-based information scans in addition to NCCT and CTA. When CTP maps are available, adding the baseline lesion mask has a detrimental effect on Dice score, reducing it by 4% ($\frac{(Dice_D - Dice_C) \times 100}{Dice_C}$); however, it still improves the rate of detection of connected components. By comparing experiment **B** with **D** and experiment **A** with **C**, we observe that additional information from the baseline CTP maps improves the final infarct prediction by 20% ($\frac{(Dice_D - Dice_B) \times 100}{Dice_B}$) and 45% ($\frac{(Dice_C - Dice_A) \times 100}{Dice_A}$) when baseline lesion mask is and is not present, respectively.

**Table 2.** Final infarct segmentation results for models *including* CTP maps. All values are averaged over the test set. 95% confidence intervals are reported. A positive volumetric difference indicates an overestimation of infarct volume compared to DWI-based ground truth. BL mask: baseline lesion mask, Exp.: experiment name. % detected CC: percentage of connected components in the ground truth that overlaps with the prediction. CTP maps include: rCBF, rCBV, MTT and TMAX.

| Exp. | Input list | Dice score ↑ | Surface Dice ↑ | Volumetric difference (ml) | Absolute volumetric difference (ml)↓ | % detected CC ↑ |
|---|---|---|---|---|---|---|
| **C** | NCCT+CTA+CTP maps | **$25.7 \pm 7.7$** | **$27.0 \pm 7.8$** | $-11.9 \pm 7.6$ | **$17.0 \pm 6.8$** | $17.0\% \pm 6.1$ |
| **D** | NCCT+CTA+CTP maps+BL mask | $24.6 \pm 7.5$ | $25.0 \pm 7.4$ | **$-8.2 \pm 9.1$** | $20.0 \pm 7.7$ | **$20.2\% \pm 7.1$** |

## 4   Discussion

We have shown that adding baseline infarct and penumbra segmentation masks improves final infarct prediction in case CTP is unavailable. In case a CTP scan is available, however, adding baseline lesion segmentation mask does not improve overlap measures. Still this addition improves the detection rate of the final infarct regions. The overall highest Dice score was obtained when the baseline CTP maps were included together with NCCT and CTA images.

The baseline lesion masks are derived from NCCT and CTA scans, which are also provided as input to the network. Although the network should theoretically be able to effectively leverage this information from NCCT and CTA alone, we observe that explicitly highlighting lesion masks as additional input improves predictions. This likely occurs because, while the network could extract this information from scans given sufficient resources, the available data is finite, making it beneficial to emphasize areas of interest. However, this improvement is no longer observed when CTP maps are included as input. This may be due to the more subtle tissue changes in baseline CT scans compared to the more discernible perfusion differences in CTP maps. Therefore, the model can identify the baseline lesion more easily and accurately from CTP maps, making the baseline lesion masks ineffective.

It should be noted that even the best-performing model has low accuracy in the final infarct prediction. One reason for this low performance is that the progression of ischemic lesions also depends on factors that occur after baseline, the most notable among which is technical treatment outcome. Not having access to this post-baseline information makes an accurate final infarct estimation difficult. Another cause that adds to the complexity of this task is a discrepancy between the input modality (CT) and the modality used for ground truth annotation (DWI). CT scans measure the radiodensity of tissue, whereas DWI measures the diffusion of water molecules within the tissue. Therefore, lesions that are visible in one modality may be absent in the other.

Optimizing performance in the prediction of the final infarct requires identifying key factors and biomarkers that influence infarct progression. Baseline imaging biomarkers are a primary source of such information. In this work, we focused on these imaging biomarkers and demonstrated the value of adding baseline lesion masks as input when CTP is unavailable. Additionally, when CTP is available, we found that combining all CTP maps with NCCT and CTA yields the most accurate final infarct prediction.

**Disclosure of Interests.** The authors have no competing interests to declare that are relevant to the content of this article.

# References

1. Back, T., Schüler, O. G.: The natural course of lesion development in brain ischemia. Springer, Vienna (2004). https://doi.org/10.1007/978-3-7091-0603-7_7
2. Birenbaum, D., Bancroft, L.W., Felsberg, G.J.: Imaging in acute stroke. West. J. Emerg. Med. **12**(1), 67–76 (2011)
3. Fahmi, F., Beenen, L.F., Streekstra, G.J., Janssen, N.Y., de Jong, H.W., Riordan, A., et al.: Head movement during CT brain perfusion acquisition of patients with

suspected acute ischemic stroke. Eur. J. Radiol. **82**, 12 (2013). https://doi.org/10.1016/j.ejrad.2013.08.039

4. Ospel, J.M., Hill, M.D., Menon, B.K., Demchuk, A., McTaggart, R., Nogueira, R., et al.: Strength of association between infarct volume and clinical outcome depends on the magnitude of infarct size: results from the ESCAPE-NA1 trial. AJNR Am. J. Neuroradiol. **42**(8), 1375–1379 (2021). https://doi.org/10.3174/ajnr.A7183

5. Gauriau, R., Bizzo, B.C., Comeau, D.S., Hillis, J.M., Bridge, C.P., Chin, J.K., et al.: Head CT deep learning model is highly accurate for early infarct estimation. Sci. Rep. **13**, 189 (2023). https://doi.org/10.1038/s41598-023-27496-5

6. Isensee, F., Jaeger, P.F., Kohl, S.A., Petersen, J., Maier-Hein, K.H.: nnU-Net: a self-configuring method for deep learning-based biomedical image segmentation. Nat. Methods **18**(2), 203–211 (2021). https://doi.org/10.1038/s41592-020-01008-z

7. de la Rosa, E., Su, R., Reyes, M., Wiest, R., Riedel, E.O., Kofler, F., et al.: ISLES'24: improving final infarct prediction in ischemic stroke using multimodal imaging and clinical data. arXiv preprint arXiv:2408.10966 (2024). https://doi.org/10.48550/arXiv.2408.10966

8. Riedel, E.O., de la Rosa, E., Baran, T.A., Petzsche, M.H., Baazaoui, H., Yang, K. et al.: ISLES 2024: The first longitudinal multimodal multi-center real-world dataset in (sub-)acute stroke. arXiv preprint arXiv:2408.11142 (2024)

# Final Stroke Infarct Segmentation Using Deep Neural Networks

Luan Matheus Trindade Dalmazo[1(✉)] and Kumaradevan Punithakumar[2]

[1] Federal University of Paraná, Curitiba, Brazil
luantrindade@ufpr.br
[2] University of Alberta, Edmonton, Canada

**Abstract.** This study aims to segment the final stroke infarct using acute stroke data. The proposed framework uses nnU-Net, one of the popular deep neural network-based algorithms for segmentation tasks. The neural network algorithm was trained using the datasets shared as a part of the ISLES'24 challenge hosted by MICCAI 2024. The performance of the trained neural network is evaluated using the Dice score, the absolute volume difference, the absolute lesion count difference, and lesion-wise F1 score. In total, seven different options for neural network training were performed and the best results were achieved through data augmentation techniques and by using only computed tomography images.

**Keywords:** Ischemic Stroke · Semantic segmentation · Neural Networks

## 1    Introduction

Ischemic stroke is a global health issue. According to the American Heart Association and the American Stroke Association, ischemic stroke is more common than hemorrhagic stroke, with 80% of those affected experiencing the ischemic type. The treatment of ischemic stroke is closely related to its early detection [1] as early identification significantly enhances the likelihood of successful treatment [2]. Image analysis is a crucial component of the clinical decision-making process. Although both magnetic resonance imaging (MRI) and computed tomography (CT) can be used, CT images are often preferred due to their speed and cost-effectiveness in the acquisition process [4].

Machine learning (ML) algorithms are increasingly employed in the detection and treatment of stroke [1], since this technology plays a crucial role in data analysis [3], enabling algorithms to contribute to the prediction, diagnosis and treatment of various diseases. ML is typically categorized into supervised and unsupervised learning. In supervised learning, models are trained on labeled data, allowing them to establish relationships between input and then generate an output. In contrast, unsupervised learning deals with unlabeled data, enabling the model to uncover hidden patterns independently.

R. Su et al. (Eds.): ISLES 2024/SWITCH 2024, LNCS 15408, pp. 95–99, 2025.
https://doi.org/10.1007/978-3-031-81101-2_11

Among supervised models, one of the most popular tasks is semantic segmentation, where each pixel in the image is classified [6]. In the medical context, nnU-Net is a state-of-the-art neural network (NN) in segmentation. This deep learning-based model proposes that segmentation could be performed automatically, allowing the network to self-configure [7].

Similar approaches were used in the last edition of the challenge, although the focus was on diffusion-weighted imaging. This paper aims to segment the final stroke infarct from preinterventional acute stroke data as part of the ISLES24 challenge. Segmentation is performed on CT images using nnU-Net, with validation metrics that include the Dice score, the absolute volume difference, the absolute lesion count difference, and the lesion-wise F1-score.

## 2   Methods

The research was carried out in two phases. The first phase focused on training the neural network, with CT images as input and binary masks representing the segmentation results as output. The second phase is dedicated to evaluating the performance of the trained model.

### 2.1   Training

The dataset was provided by ISLES'24 [8,9] and includes preprocessed images, clinical information, and raw images. The modalities present are CT and MRI, totaling 150 patient data samples. Training was performed as each batch became available: the first batch contained 46 patient data, the second 47, and the last 57. Initially, training was conducted using only images from each respective batch. However, after the sixth training, data augmentation techniques such as random rotation, noise addition, and flipping were adopted.

A Python script was used to align with the nnU-Net structure. The preprocessing phase, managed by the model, involved collecting foreground class intensities and calculating the mean and standard deviation. Normalization was applied to all training images before they were input into the neural network.

The training was performed with the default nnU-Net settings for 1000 epochs. At the end of the training, the next phase is prediction, where an image is input to the network, and the output is the segmented mask. Figure 1 illustrates the pipeline used for the training.

### 2.2   Evaluation

The evaluation will be conducted considering the following metrics:

- Dice Score: Similarity and overlap between the ground truth and the generated segmentation.
- Absolute Volume Difference: Volumetric difference between the ground truth and the NN output.

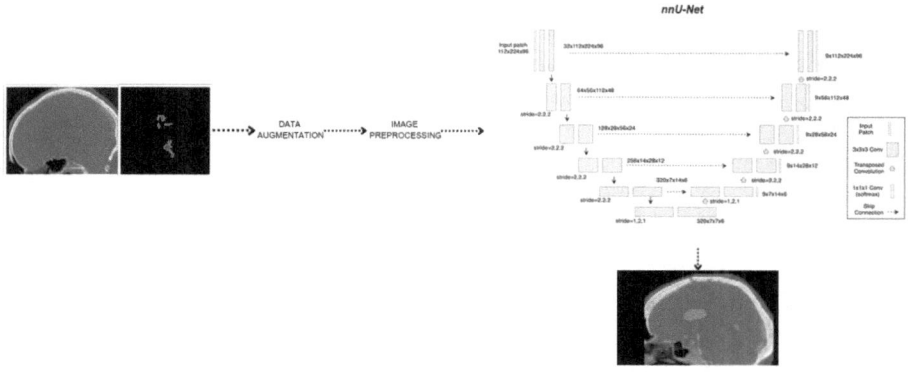

**Fig. 1.** Overview of the machine learning pipeline used for segmentation.

- Absolute Lesion Count Difference: Absolute difference in the number of lesions found in the model's output compared to the ground truth.
- Lesion-wise F1-Score: Evaluation of the algorithm's performance per lesion using a combination of precision and recall.

## 3   Results

In total, seven trainings were conducted. Table 1 illustrates the best Dice score obtained for each model with its respective configuration. This result was obtained through the report generated by nnU-Net itself. 20% of the sets were allocated by nnunet as the validation set, and three additional sets were assigned manually to calculate the metrics for the best model.

**Table 1.** Best Dice score obtained for each model and its configuration

| Position | Dice Score | Best Configuration |
|---|---|---|
| First | 0.2171 | 3D Cascade Full Resolution |
| Second | 0.1975 | 3D Full Resolution |
| Third | 0.1591 | 3D Full Resolution |
| Fourth | 0.1600 | 3D Full Resolution |
| Fifth | 0.1617 | 3D Full Resolution |
| **Sixth** | **0.3407** | **Combination of 3D Low Resolution and Cascade Full Resolution** |
| Seventh | 0.3020 | Combination of 3D Low Resolution and Cascade Full Resolution |

Table 2 illustrates the types of images used, the techniques employed, and the number of inputs. Training sessions were conducted as new datasets became

**Table 2.** Types of images used, techniques employed, and number of inputs

| Position | Number of Inputs | Images and Techniques |
|---|---|---|
| First | 46 | CTA, perfusion-maps, no data augmentation |
| Second | 93 | CTA, perfusion-maps, no data augmentation |
| Third | 93 | CTA, perfusion-maps, without header and no data augmentation |
| Fourth | 93 | CTA, perfusion-maps and CTP, without header and no data augmentation |
| Fifth | 93 | CTA, no data augmentation |
| **Sixth** | **299** | **CTA, data augmentation** |
| Seventh | 299 | CTA (raw and preprocessed), data augmentation and without header |

available. For each training session, different combinations of modalities and techniques were tested.

The results for the metrics assessed for the best model were evaluated using the inference script provided by the challenge organizers. A validation set was proposed, and Table 3 illustrates the metrics for the best model.

**Table 3.** Metrics assessed for the best model

| Metric | Value |
|---|---|
| Dice Score | 0.5743 |
| Absolute Volume Difference | 1.599 ml |
| Absolute Lesion Count Difference | 6.0 |
| Lesion-wise F1 Score | 0.2645 |

At the time of writing of this paper, the results for the metrics evaluated in the *Final Test Phase Leaderboard* had not yet been released. Therefore, the tests were conducted using images from the training set.

## 4   Discussion and Conclusion

The results indicate that the data augmentation technique was effective in improving the Dice score and that the CT modality was the most effective in achieving good results. Throughout the training sessions, it was observed that the number of inputs had a direct impact on the model performance; in the later sessions, the inclusion of 299 inputs (the number of preprocessed CT images) positively affected the prediction quality.

To apply the header removal technique, a Python script was used. The initial idea was to remove the header and then reapply it during prediction. However, the removal of this information had a negative impact, suggesting that the information present in the image is important for learning.

The use of raw and preprocessed data also impacted the final result. The combination of raw and modified data reduced the model's overall Dice score.

Therefore, the best model utilized only preprocessed CT images. It is understood that raw data contains noise that can negatively influence the network's training.

Model improvement can be achieved through data augmentation, and further enhancements can be made by refining the framework configuration for this segmentation task. This includes adjusting the batch size to allow the model to process more data during each training session and experimenting with different loss functions, which can have a significant impact; in this case, a combination of Dice score and cross-entropy was used. The results are expected to highlight the complexity of segmenting the final stroke infarct using acute stroke data and provide valuable suggestions for further improvements in the model's training process.

**Acknowledgments.** This work was carried out with the support of Fundação Araucária/SETI, the Federal University of Paraná, the Mitacs Globalink Research Internship Program, and the University of Alberta.

**Disclosure of Interests.** The authors have no competing interests to declare.

# References

1. Ruksakulpiwat, S., Phianhasin, L., Benjasirisan, C., Schiltz, N.K.: Using neural networks algorithm in ischemic stroke diagnosis: a systematic review. J. Multidiscip. Healthc. **16**, 2593–2602 (2023). https://doi.org/10.2147/JMDH.S421280
2. O'Connell, G.C., Walsh, K.B., Smothers, C.G., et al.: Use of deep artificial neural networks to identify stroke during triage via subtle changes in circulating cell counts. BMC Neurol. **22**, 206 (2022). https://doi.org/10.1186/s12883-022-02726-x
3. Sarker, I.H.: Machine learning: algorithms, real-world applications and research directions. SN Comput. Sci. **2**(3), 160 (2021). https://doi.org/10.1007/s42979-021-00592-x
4. Pereira, D.R., Filho, P.P.R., de Rosa, G.H., Papa, J.P., Albuquerque, V.H.C.: Stroke lesion detection using convolutional neural networks. In: 2018 International Joint Conference on Neural Networks (IJCNN), Rio de Janeiro, Brazil (2018), pp. 1–6 (2018). https://doi.org/10.1109/IJCNN.2018.8489199
5. Jiang, T., Gradus, J.L., Rosellini, A.J.: Supervised machine learning: a brief primer. Behav. Ther. **51**(5), 675–687 (2020). https://doi.org/10.1016/j.beth.2020.05.002
6. Hao, S., Zhou, Y., Guo, Y.: A brief survey on semantic segmentation with deep learning. Neurocomputing **406**, 302–321 (2020). https://doi.org/10.1016/j.neucom.2019.11.118
7. Isensee, F., Jaeger, P.F., Kohl, S.A.A., et al.: nnU-Net: a self-configuring method for deep learning-based biomedical image segmentation. Nat. Methods **18**, 203–211 (2021). https://doi.org/10.1038/s41592-020-01008-z
8. de la Rosa, E., et al.: ISLES'24: Improving final infarct prediction in ischemic stroke using multimodal imaging and clinical data. *arXiv preprint* arXiv:2408.10966. Retrieved from https://arxiv.org/abs/2408.10966 (2024)
9. Riedel, E.O., et al.: ISLES 2024: The first longitudinal multimodal multi-center real-world dataset in (sub-)acute stroke. arXiv preprint arXiv:2408.11142. Retrieved from https://arxiv.org/abs/2408.11142 (2024)

# A Multi-modal Deep Learning Framework for Final Infarct Prediction in Acute Ischemic Stroke: Combining CTA, NCCT, and Clinical Data

Eneko Uruñuela[1(✉)], Annabella Bregazzi[1], and Matthias Wilms[1,2,3,4]

[1] Department of Radiology, University of Calgary, Calgary, AB, Canada
eneko.urunuela@ucalgary.ca
[2] Hotchkiss Brain Institute, University of Calgary, Calgary, Canada
[3] Alberta Children's Hospital Research Institute, University of Calgary, Calgary, Canada
[4] Departments of Pediatrics and Community Health Sciences, University of Calgary, Calgary, Canada

**Abstract.** Timely treatment decisions facilitate optimal outcomes in acute ischemic stroke patients, wherein computed tomography (CT) imaging data represents the primary imaging modality used for initial clinical assessment. This study presents and evaluates a novel deep learning architecture that integrates non-contrast computed tomography (NCCT) images, CT angiography (CTA) images, and mean and maximum projections of the CTA images, along with clinical data for tissue outcome predictions in patients with acute ischemic stroke. The proposed model is based on a convolutional neural network (CNN), including an encoder module, multiple fully connected layers, and a decoder. We trained and evaluated the proposed deep learning model using data from the ISLES 2024 challenge, which included 150 patients, of which we allocated 80% for training and 20% for evaluation. The evaluation showed that our model achieved a mean Dice score of 0.04 ($\pm 0.07$), a mean absolute volume difference of 35 ml ($\pm 24.7$ ml), a mean lesion count difference of 207 ($\pm 28.65$), and a mean lesion-wise F1 score of 0.13 ($\pm 0.15$). While our model overestimated the size of small infarct cores, its satisfactory performance detecting larger lesions highlights the potential of simple and widely-available CTA images and its mean and maximum projections, along with the NCCT data and relevant clinical information for predicting final infarct brain tissue in patients with acute ischemic stroke.

**Keywords:** CTA · Stroke · Final Infarct Prediction · Deep Learning

## 1 Introduction

Stroke is a cerebrovascular disorder characterized by the sudden interruption of arterial blood flow, leading to compromised cerebral perfusion and potentially-irreversible damage to brain tissue in the affected parenchyma [3]. Due to the

R. Su et al. (Eds.): ISLES 2024/SWITCH 2024, LNCS 15408, pp. 100–105, 2025.
https://doi.org/10.1007/978-3-031-81101-2_12

resulting neuronal injury, acute ischemic stroke (AIS) represents a leading cause of prolonged disability, morbidity, and mortality [5]. Consequently, timely diagnosis and treatment of subtle clinical manifestations are crucial to achieve the best possible outcomes for patients with AIS who present early enough to save the brain tissue affected by the hypoperfusion but not yet infarcted [5,19].

The diagnosis, assessment, and treatment planning, including triage to a tertiary center, of patients with AIS depends heavily on neuroimaging data. Within this context, computed tomography (CT) is the most commonly used imaging modality in centers world-wide due to its rapid acquisition time and widespread availability in emergency rooms [6]. More precisely, non-contrast CT (NCCT) is mainly employed in the acute phase at admission to differentiate between various stroke sub-types and to rule out other causes, such as hemorrhages. Additionally, CT angiography (CTA) is frequently utilized to obtain knowledge about the collateral situation and clot location, while CT perfusion (CTP) is often used to obtain knowledge about the extent of the ischemic core and the salvageable penumbra [8,9,15]. To guide treatment decisions in patients with AIS, the prediction of tissue outcomes for various treatment options has sparked considerable interest in recent years. Briefly described, these methods use imaging and clinical data obtained in the acute phase after patient admission to predict the expected tissue outcome for different treatment outcomes [18]. CTP imaging data has been used in most cases for this purpose, either using derived perfusion maps or the full CTP imaging data [2]. However, CTP may not be available in all primary care centers due to the license fees and technical expertise required for its acquisition. Moreover, CTP is known to be prone to motion artefacts and expose patients to considerable ionizing radiation. Recently, machine learning models that integrate only NCCT and CTA images have been shown to yield results consistent with those predicted by a model based on CTP imaging [16], underscoring the potential of these simpler modalities. Furthermore, integrating readily-available clinical information such as sex and age has recently been shown to improve some aspects of deep learning-based tissue outcome prediction [1]. Therefore, tissue outcome prediction methods employing machine learning methodologies based on NCCT and CTA imaging alongside clinical variables could facilitate improved treatment decision in primary care centers [4,17].

The aim of this work was to develop, evaluate, and explore the feasibility of a novel deep learning architecture that integrates information from widely available NCCT and CTA images with clinical data to predict tissue outcomes in patients with AIS. The proposed model was specifically evaluated using data from the Ischemic Stroke Lesion Segmentation (ISLES) 2024 challenge [11].

## 2   Methods

### 2.1   Dataset and Preprocessing

The proposed method was trained and evaluated using the provided preprocessed CTA images (which were registered to the NCCT images), raw NCCT images, and clinical data from 150 patients with AIS from the ISLES 2024 challenge [11,12]. Two patients without clinical data were excluded. The data was further preprocessed to ensure that all images exhibited consistent voxel spacing and image sizes. Therefore, all images were resampled to a uniform voxel spacing of $0.45 \times 0.45 \times 2.0$ mm using a linear interpolation. Then, skullstripping was performed for the NCCT and the CTA images using simple intensity-based thresholding between 1 and 100 HU. Afterwards, cropping and zero-padding was applied within the axial plane so that the brain tissue of each image was centered with a consistent size of $416 \times 416$ voxels. Next, the mean and maximum projections of the CTA images were calculated at the voxel level [10]. The mean projection was calculated by averaging the voxel values of the CTA images using a sliding window approach along the z-axis, with a width of 5 slices. Similarly, the maximum projection was determined using the maximum voxel value within each 5-slice window. Finally, the four images were independently normalized to have a mean of zero and a standard deviation of one. From the available clinical variables, we extracted and used those which have shown utility in previous tissue outcome prediction works: age, NIHSS score at admission, mRS score at admission, sex, atrial fibrillation, hypertension, and diabetes [1].

## 2.2 Model Architecture

The proposed CNN model was trained using the following set of four distinct patient-wise input images organized as separate channels within the input tensor: the NCCT image, the CTA image, and both the mean and maximum projections of the CTA images (see Sect. 2.1). Given the varying number of axial slices of the patients' images, we developed the model to predict final infarcts in a slice-by-slice manner (*i.e.,* in 2D) using the following three-module architecture (illustrated in Fig. 1):

1. **CNN encoder:** The input NCCT, CTA, mean projected CTA, and maximum projected CTA are processed by the CNN encoder. This encoder is

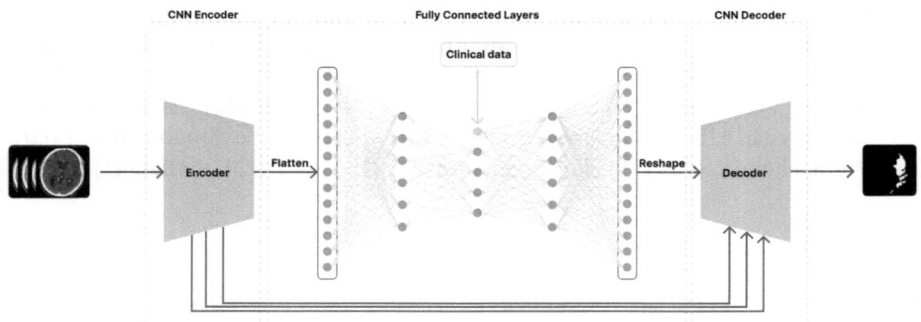

**Fig. 1.** Overview of the proposed model consisting of a CNN encoder, a series of fully connected layers, and a CNN decoder.

organized into three levels, each containing two internal blocks. More precisely, each block consists of two convolutional layers that utilize $3 \times 3$ kernels and rectified linear unit (ReLU) activations. Following these layers, a 2D max-pooling layer is employed to reduce the spatial resolution of the original images, applying a kernel size of $2 \times 2$ with a stride of 2.

2. **Fully connected layers:** The fully connected layers function as an intermediary between the CNN encoder and decoder in our proposed architecture. This module integrates the high-level image representations acquired by the encoder with pertinent clinical data while also incorporating a global spatial context across modalities. More specifically, the module comprises of four fully connected layers: the first two layers reduce the dimensionality of the embeddings and employ ReLU activations. The last two layers incorporate the clinical information described in Sect. 2.1 by injecting it into the embeddings vector and up-sample the embeddings to the size required by the CNN decoder module, which mimics the encoder module described above.

3. **CNN decoder:** The reshaped two-dimensional embeddings matrix is then processed by the CNN decoder. The CNN decoder is responsible for restoring the original spatial resolution by upsampling the feature representations. Therefore, the decoder essentially mirrors the encoder blocks. Additionally, at each level, the output from the encoder is concatenated with the output of the decoder's up-sampling layer via skip connections. The final layer of the decoder consists of a convolutional layer followed by a softmax layer. Finally, a threshold of 0.5 is used to compute the binary final infarct mask based on the probability maps generated by the CNN.

### 2.3   Model Training

Python and PyTorch were used for model development, which was trained and tested using an NVIDIA GeForce RTX 3090 with 24 GB of memory optimizing the Dice loss function [14]. Practically, 80% of the data were used for training while the remaining 20% were used for testing. Only slices that contained a stroke lesion were used for training the CNN while all slices (*i.e.,* including non-lesion slices) were considered when testing the model on unseen data. The final model was trained using 100 epochs, a batch size of 8 with an initial learning rate of 0.0001 and using the Adam optimizer with a step-based learning rate decay. Overall, the total number of trainable parameters in the model was 83,551,774.

## 3   Results: Model Testing

We evaluated the proposed CNN model using several quantitative metrics provided by the ISLES 24 challenge organizers using *panoptica* [7]. Therefore, all quantitative metrics were calculated for each patient's 3D images and averaged for the full test set. Quantitatively, the proposed CNN model led to a mean Dice score of 0.04 ($\pm 0.07$), an average absolute volume difference of 35 ml ($\pm 24.7$ ml), a mean lesion count difference of 207 ($\pm 28.65$), and a mean lesion-specific

F1-score of 0.13 ($\pm$0.15). A qualitative evaluation revealed that the model over-predicted the lesion tissue in cases where the final infarct lesions were small, but accurately predicted larger lesions.

## 4   Discussion

In this work, we evaluated the feasibility and effectiveness of our proposed CNN model for predicting final infarcts in patients with AIS. This model integrates NCCT, CTA, and both mean and maximum projections of CTA, alongside relevant clinical data. We trained and tested our model using the dataset provided by the ISLES 2024 challenge. Our results demonstrate that our multimodal model struggled with accurately predicting small final infarct lesions in patients with AIS, while performing adequately on larger lesions. These results align with previous studies showing that models that rely on CTA images overpredict the infarct core, especially when the CTA images are obtained using rapid acquisition protocols [13, 20]. This discrepancy may be attributed to the fact that these CTA images are more heavily weighted towards vascular blood flow rather than blood volume [13]. Unfortunately, we could not determine whether lack of accuracy of our model was affected by the timing of CTA acquisition since this information was not provided with the ISLES 2024 challenge data.

While our proposed model benefits from using widely available and accessible data, which makes it practically relevant, incorporating temporal data in the form of CTP images could improve the model's ability to predict the final tissue outcome. Within this context, the spatio-temporal patterns related to blood flow and volume in CTP datasets have been shown to be particularly beneficial for predicting final infarcts in patients with AIS [2]. Thus, an ensemble architecture integrating the spatio-temporal information derived from perfusion CT with the model presented here may yield more robust and accurate results. Additionally, conducting ablation studies will be essential to understand the contribution of each input feature and to assess their individual impact on model performance.

**Acknowledgments.** This study was funded by the Alberta Innovates postdoctoral fellowship program and the Heart and Stroke foundation (G-24-0037894).

**Disclosure of Interests.** The authors have no competing interests to declare that are relevant to the content of this article.

## References

1. Amador, K., Gutierrez, A., Winder, A., Fiehler, J., Wilms, M., Forkert, N.D.: Providing clinical context to the spatio-temporal analysis of 4D CT perfusion to predict acute ischemic stroke lesion outcomes. J. Biomed. Inform. **149**, 104567 (2024). https://doi.org/10.1016/j.jbi.2023.104567
2. Amador, K., et al.: Hybrid spatio-temporal transformer network for predicting ischemic stroke lesion outcomes from 4D CT perfusion imaging. Med. Image Comput. Comput. Assist. Interv. - MICCAI **2022**, 644–654 (2022). https://doi.org/10.1007/978-3-031-16437-8_62

3. Donnan, G.A., et al.: Secondary prevention of stroke. Lancet **372**(9643), 1036 (2008). https://doi.org/10.1016/s0140-6736(08)61439-7
4. Feng, R., et al.: Deep learning guided stroke management: a review of clinical applications. J. NeuroInterventional Surg. **10**(4), 358–362 (2017). https://doi.org/10.1136/neurintsurg-2017-013355
5. Furlan, A.J.: Time is brain. Stroke **37**(12), 2863–2864 (2006). https://doi.org/10.1161/01.str.0000251852.07152.63
6. Handschu, R., et al.: Acute stroke management in the local general hospital. Stroke **32**(4), 866–870 (2001). https://doi.org/10.1161/01.str.32.4.866
7. Kofler, F., et al.: Panoptica – instance-wise evaluation of 3D semantic and instance segmentation maps (2023). https://doi.org/10.48550/ARXIV.2312.02608
8. Ma, H., et al.: Thrombolysis guided by perfusion imaging up to 9 hours after onset of stroke. N. Engl. J. Med. **380**(19), 1795–1803 (2019). https://doi.org/10.1056/nejmoa1813046
9. Nogueira, R.G., et al.: Thrombectomy 6 to 24 hours after stroke with a mismatch between deficit and infarct. N. Engl. J. Med. **378**(1), 11–21 (2018). https://doi.org/10.1056/nejmoa1706442
10. Palsson, F., et al.: Prediction of tissue outcome in acute ischemic stroke based on single-phase CT angiography at admission. Front. Neurol. **15** (Mar 2024). https://doi.org/10.3389/fneur.2024.1330497
11. Riedel, E.O., et al.: Isles 2024: the first longitudinal multimodal multi-center real-world dataset in (sub-)acute stroke (2024). https://doi.org/10.48550/ARXIV.2408.11142
12. de la Rosa, E., et al.: Isles'24: improving final infarct prediction in ischemic stroke using multimodal imaging and clinical data (2024). https://doi.org/10.48550/ARXIV.2408.10966
13. Sharma, M., et al.: CT angiographic source images: flow- or volume-weighted? Am. J. Neuroradiol. **32**(2), 359–364 (2010). https://doi.org/10.3174/ajnr.a2282
14. Sudre, C.H., et al.: Generalised Dice Overlap as a Deep Learning Loss Function for Highly Unbalanced Segmentations, pp. 240–248. Springer International Publishing (2017). https://doi.org/10.1007/978-3-319-67558-9_28
15. Thomalla, G., et al.: MRI-guided thrombolysis for stroke with unknown time of onset. N. Engl. J. Med. **379**(7), 611–622 (2018). https://doi.org/10.1056/nejmoa1804355
16. Wang, C., et al.: Deep learning-based identification of acute ischemic core and deficit from non-contrast CT and CTA (2021). https://doi.org/10.25384/SAGE.C.5461480.V1
17. Winder, A.J., et al.: Challenges and potential of artificial intelligence in neuroradiology. Clin. Neuroradiol. **34**(2), 293–305 (2024). https://doi.org/10.1007/s00062-024-01382-7
18. Yedavalli, V.S., et al.: Artificial intelligence in stroke imaging: current and future perspectives. Clin. Imaging **69**, 246–254 (2021). https://doi.org/10.1016/j.clinimag.2020.09.005
19. del Zoppo, G.J., et al.: Expansion of the time window for treatment of acute ischemic stroke with intravenous tissue plasminogen activator: a science advisory from the American heart association/American stroke association. Stroke **40**(8), 2945–2948 (2009). https://doi.org/10.1161/strokeaha.109.192535
20. Öman, O., et al.: 3D convolutional neural networks applied to ct angiography in the detection of acute ischemic stroke. Eur. Radiol. Exp. **3**(1), 1–11 (2019). https://doi.org/10.1186/s41747-019-0085-6

# Author Index

R. Su et al. (Eds.): ISLES 2024/SWITCH 2024, LNCS 15408, pp. 107–108, 2025.
https://doi.org/10.1007/978-3-031-81101-2

# Organization

## SWITCH Organizing Committee

| | |
|---|---|
| Ewout Heylen | KU Leuven, Belgium |
| Richard McKinley | Inselspital Bern, Switzerland |
| Frank te Nijenhuis | Erasmus MC, The Netherlands |
| Leonhard Rist | Friedrich-Alexander-Universität Erlangen-Nürnberg, Germany |
| Ezequiel de la Rosa | University of Zurich, Switzerland |
| Danny Ruijters | Eindhoven University of Technology, The Netherlands |
| Markus D. Schirmer | Massachusetts General Hospital, Harvard Medical School, USA |
| Ruisheng Su | Eindhoven University of Technology, The Netherlands |
| Theo van Walsum | Erasmus MC, The Netherlands |
| Susanne Wegener | University Hospital Zurich, Switzerland |
| Roland Wiest | Inselspital Bern, Switzerland |

## ISLES Organizing Committee

| | |
|---|---|
| Jan S. Kirschke | Klinikum rechts der Isar, Technical University of Munich, Germany |
| Bjoern Menze | University of Zurich, Switzerland |
| Mauricio Reyes | University of Bern, Switzerland |
| Ezequiel de la Rosa | University of Zurich, Switzerland |
| Ruisheng Su | Eindhoven University of Technology, The Netherlands |
| Susanne Wegener | University Hospital Zurich, Switzerland |
| Roland Wiest | Inselspital Bern, Switzerland |
| Benedikt Wiestler | Klinikum rechts der Isar, Technical University of Munich, Germany |